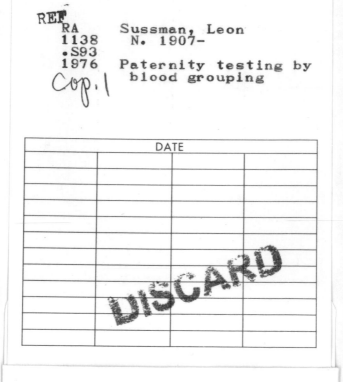

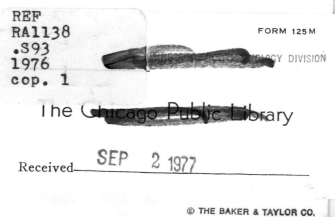

# Paternity Testing
# By Blood Grouping

*Second Edition*

# Paternity Testing
# By Blood Grouping

*By*

LEON N. SUSSMAN, M.D.

*Attending Hematologist and Director of Blood Bank*
*Beth Israel Medical Center*
*Clinical Professor of Medicine, Mount Sinai School of*
*Medicine of the City University of New York*
*New York, New York*

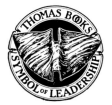

CHARLES C THOMAS · PUBLISHER
*Springfield · Illinois · U.S.A.*

*Published and Distributed Throughout the World by*

CHARLES C THOMAS • PUBLISHER

Bannerstone House

301-327 East Lawrence Avenue, Springfield, Illinois, U.S.A.

ISBN 0-398-03523-7

Library of Congress Catalog Card Number 75-37503

*With THOMAS BOOKS careful attention is given to all details of
manufacturing and design. It is the Publisher's desire to present books that
are satisfactory as to their physical qualities and artistic possibilities and
appropriate for their particular use. THOMAS BOOKS will be true to those
laws of quality that assure a good name and good will.*

First Edition *(Blood Grouping Tests)* © 1968

Second Edition © 1976

*Printed in the United States of America*

*C-1*

**Library of Congress Cataloging in Publication Data**

Sussman, Leon N.   1907-
  Paternity testing by blood grouping.
  First ed. published in 1968 under title: Blood
grouping tests.
  Includes bibliographies and index.
  1. Paternity testing. 2. Blood groups. 3. Forensic
hematology. I. Title. [DNLM: 1. Blood groups.
2. Forensic medicine. 3. Paternity. QY415 S964b]
RA1138.S93 1976       614'.19       75-37503
ISBN 0-398-03523-7

TO
EVELYN

# CONTRIBUTORS

**Dale Dykes, A.B.:** Research Associate, Minneapolis War Memorial Blood Bank, Minneapolis, Minnesota.

**Angelyn A. Konugres, Ph.D.:** Director of Blood Bank, Boston Hospital for Women; Principal Associate in Obstetrics and Gynecology, Harvard Medical School; Director of Research, Boston Hospital for Women.

**Byron A. Myhre, M.D., Ph.D.:** Professor of Pathology; Head of Immunopathology; UCLA School of Medicine, Harbor General Hospital Campus, California.

**Herbert Polesky, M.D.:** Director, Minneapolis War Memorial Blood Bank, Minneapolis, Minnesota; Associate Professor, Department of Pathology and Laboratory Medicine, University of Minnesota.

**Alexander S. Wiener, M.D.:** Professor, Department of Forensic Medicine, New York University School of Medicine, New York City.

# PREFACE

**To the First Edition**

THE SCIENCE OF BLOOD grouping has expanded so rapidly in the past twenty years, and publications related to this subject have so flooded the literature, that the newcomers in the field can well flounder in the seeming chaos. The purpose of this book is to attempt an orderly account of the theoretical principles, followed by practical technical details of the procedures used. The actual application of the findings, both theoretical and practical, to the problems in clinical and medicolegal situations will be demonstrated. A visionary approach to the future usefulness will be attempted with full realization of the risks of this presumption in such an actively advancing specialty.

The number of totally independent blood group systems, each of which divides blood into several independent subgroups, combine to make the complete blood typing of a person an extremely individual characteristic. At the present time at least 50,000,000 individuals can be clearly differentiated by blood typing. It is estimated that except for identical twins, there are no two persons with exactly the same detailed blood grouping. It is indeed fortunate for the human race that only a few of these differences are of significance in blood transfusions, or it would be almost impossible to find a "compatible" donor. On the other hand, it is the great individuality that makes blood grouping so invaluable in paternity studies, personal identification, and other medicolegal applications.

The field of blood grouping demands absolute accuracy on the part of the technician as well as the doctor. In no other branch of medicine is error so catastrophic, since the life of a patient may be jeopardized by inattention or inaccuracy. In the medicolegal aspect, errors may invoke miscarriages of justice, cause disruption of families, stigmatize children, and cast doubt on the reliability of the entire field of blood grouping tests. A ritual of checking and rechecking has developed, with each step controlled by reactions between known cells and serums. A complete knowledge of the technical pitfalls is essential. Of equal importance is a thorough familiarity with all the theoretically possible variations and exceptions that can occur. Thus, a thoroughly knowledgeable expert working under the best of physical conditions and with the most reliable serums is able to obtain reproducible results. Such results can then be interpreted with security and permit valid, reliable conclusions. It is this combination of knowledge, training, dedication, and understanding that has resulted in the absolute accuracy that this science demands. And it is to maintain these high standards that, it is hoped, this book will prove helpful.

# PREFACE

## To the Second Edition

T HE USEFULNESS of blood grouping tests in solving medicolegal problems has advanced far beyond the present meager reports which emanated from the Medicolegal Committee of the American Medical Association in 1960. The knowledgeable serologist engaged in blood grouping should not feel hampered by the restrictions which limits his tests to only the A-B-O, M-N, and Rh-Hr systems.

In this edition, the reader will find valuable contributions which enlarge the A-B-O system by the study of the subgroup of A; the M-N system by the new findings of the S, s, and $S^u$ factors; and the Rh-Hr system by the use of anti-hr(f) and by the means of excluding deleted genes and unusual exceptions. In addition the availability of antisera for the testing of the Kell, Kidd, Duffy, Lutheran, $Xg^a$, and other systems indicate the approach to maturity of these genetically dependent blood groups.

The preview of the future, expressed in the first edition has now been brought closer to reality by the illuminating chapter on erythrocyte isoenzymes and plasma proteins. The technics for these tests can quickly be mastered and will add considerably to the maximum contribution forensic science can make to the exclusion of a falsely accused man. An additional chapter discusses the probability of paternity where no exclusion can be demonstrated. Based on blood group statistics, this chapter further presents the inherent dangers in such conclusions.

These basic accomplishments can be adapted to the many other aspects of medicolegal problems, such as kidnapped children, personal identification, and inheritance disputes. Knowledge, understanding, training, and dedication are essential for the absolute accuracy demanded of this area of forensic pathology. Required as well, is the constant awareness of the new contributions to this ever growing field.

# ACKNOWLEDGMENTS

I AM EVERLASTINGLY indebted to my wife, Evelyn, for her expert proofreading as well as her patience and endurance during the writing of this book. I am also greatly indebted to Mrs. Hannah Pretshold for her assistance in the research and in the preparation of the bibliography, and to Mrs. Irene Whitestone for her careful preparation of the manuscript. I also want to take this opportunity to express my deep appreciation to Susan and Monte Hurowitz for their generous support and to Dr. A. S. Wiener who again was most lavish with his time, advice, and assistance.

The cooperation of the coauthors, Dr. Byron A. Myhre, Dr. Angelyn A. Konugres, Dr. Herbert Polesky, Mr. Dale Dykes, and Dr. Alexander S. Wiener has added immeasurably to the value of this book by the contribution of their expertise.

L.N.S.

# CONTENTS

# Paternity Testing
# By Blood Grouping

CHAPTER ONE

# GENERAL CONSIDERATIONS

Leon N. Sussman

## HISTORICAL DEVELOPMENT

IT WAS KARL LANDSTEINER, later to be named the "Father of Immunohematology," who first reported the agglutination of human red blood cells by the serum of blood obtained from other humans. By this observation, he discovered the first three blood groups subsequently called A, B, and O.[1, 2] The fourth and rarest blood group, later to be called AB, was described shortly thereafter by Decastello and Sturli.[3] It was shown that the antigen determining the blood group was on the red blood cells, and the reciprocal antibody against the antigen missing from the red blood cells was present in the serum. Thus, the A person had anti-**B** in the serum, the B person had anti-**A** in the serum, the O person had both anti-**A** and anti-**B** in the serum, while the AB person had neither anti-**A** nor anti-**B** in the serum.* With this information, the blood type of a person could be determined by testing the red blood cells with known anti-**A** serum and anti-**B** serum and the blood group confirmed by testing the serum with known group A cells and group B cells.

Widespread scientific interest and research soon followed this discovery, and the next few years saw many publications relating to the human blood groups. Epstein and Ottenberg,[4] in 1908, suggested that the A-B-O blood groups were inherited characteristics. In 1901, von Dungern and Hirszfeld[5] carried the studies further, postulating that the blood groups are inherited in accordance with the Mendelian laws by two pairs of allelic genes *A-a* and *B-b*. In 1924, Bernstein[6] explained the inheritance of the

---

* Symbols for blood factors (serological specificities) and their corresponding antibodies are printed in boldface type, symbols for agglutinogens and phenotypes in regular type, while symbols for genes and genotypes are printed in italics.

A-B-O blood group by the presently accepted theory of multiple allelic genes, and used population genetics to prove that the theories of Dungern and Hirszfeld were incorrect. Wiener[7] in his classic book, *Blood Groups and Transfusion,* collected over 10,000 such family studies; Andresen in 1947 reported 20,000 mother-child tests,[8] and many other authors have contributed sizable family studies to reinforce Bernstein's theory of the inheritance of the A-B-O blood groups by multiple allelic genes.[9]

With this precedent and example, the study of all other blood group systems was provided with a model of procedure. As other systems were discovered, they were promptly tested and found to conform to the Mendelian laws of heredity. Resulting from this widespread investigation of family studies in large numbers—the proof of inheritance, the immutable nature of genetically determined blood grouping and the reliability of the testing methods—all were established. In spite of many publications dealing with superficially appearing deviations from the established laws of inheritance, none of these disturbed the essential facts. Each modification noted, whether genetic or acquired, served only to fortify the laws. Each variation required explanation within the laws; either by the effect of modifying genes, unusual inheritance, or illegitimacy. Occasionally and most lamentably, they could only be explained by technical error or lack of knowledge.

As intensive investigation of the A-B-O system was pursued, it was only natural that other differences in human blood should be sought. This led Landsteiner and Levine[10] in 1927 to describe serums, obtained from rabbits immunized by the injection of human red blood cells that differentiated between samples of red blood cells in a manner unrelated to the A-B-O blood group system. To the new blood group system they assigned the symbols M-N, from the word iMmuNe, and explained the inheritance of the M-N types by a two-gene system. Thus, a sample of red blood cells could be agglutinated by anti-**M** and/or anti-**N** serum. People could then be divided by the reaction of their red blood cells with these two antiserums into M, N, and MN types. The mode of inheritance of the genes determining these types was strictly Mendelian as proved again by large numbers of family studies.

Confirmation of these findings and conclusions came quickly from several other workers including Schiff[11] and Wiener and Vaisberg.[12]

Another by-product of the M-N experiment was the discovery by Landsteiner and Levine of an additional antiserum which could distinguish two separate groups of blood samples. This system was given the name P by the discoverers who described the inheritance as also following Mendelian laws.[13] The further clarification of this system was delayed until 1955 when Sanger[14] identified the Tj[a] antigen as part of the P system. To date, the P system is of little clinical significance and has not been of great value in medicolegal studies because of indistinct reactions and weak antiserums which lessen reliability.

The greatest stimulus to the field of blood grouping took place in 1940 with the discovery of the Rh factor by Landsteiner and Wiener.[15] The impact of the relationship of this factor to intragroup transfusion reactions (described by Wiener and Peters[16]) and to erythroblastosis fetalis (described by Levine, Katzin, Vogel, and Burnham[17, 18, 19]) was such as to create an entire new science —immunohematology.

The complexities of the Rh system were so thoroughly investigated that in the next few years at least 500 separate publications appeared on this subject alone. Laboratories and investigators from many lands began to search into the newly discovered world of blood groups. The advent of World War II and the increased use of blood for transfusions made available tremendous research material. Soon more individual differences in blood could be demonstrated with new blood group systems independent of previously described systems. Subgroups of the M-N system such as **S-s** were reported.[20, 21] Rapidly thereafter, the Kell-Cellano (**K-k**),[22, 23] **Lewis,**[24] **Lutheran,**[25] **Duffy,**[26] **Kidd,**[27] **Diego,**[28] **Vel,**[29] and many others were discovered and were added to the list of public (major) or private (minor) blood group systems. The more recent addition of the genetically determined polymorphism of the various blood proteins and erythrocyte enzymes have greatly expanded this list of individual characteristics. Closer and closer has this science come to fulfilling Landsteiner's prophesy that the individuality of blood will someday be comparable to the individuality of fingerprints.

## MEDICOLEGAL APPLICATIONS

### Principles

The study of the blood group systems concerned itself not only with the individual differences between blood samples but also with the rigid obedience of the inheritance of these differences to the laws of genetics. Family trees could be constructed demonstrating the passage of each blood factor from the preceding to the succeeding generation whenever samples could be obtained for testing. Little time was lost in applying these reliable, easily performed tests to problems involving filial relationships as in parentage studies for paternity and maternity, "mixed baby" problems in nurseries, stolen baby and kidnapping cases, immigration and citizenship claims, and in problems of estatology, anthropology, and personal identification. Criminology utilized this new science in the identification of blood types from blood stains and body secretions. Saliva, sputum, sweat, nasal secretion, seminal stains, and even urine have been typed; and the resulting information compared with the blood grouping findings of suspects and victims. Since results of blood grouping tests are of value primarily in a negative way—that is to prove that specimens are *not* identical—the elimination of noninvolved persons may be achieved. Thus, forensic medicine acquired a most valuable tool.

These manifold applications of blood grouping tests were made possible by the great restraint of the early workers who insisted on attention to details of procedures and continuous monitoring of all reactions with known cells and serums as controls. Their reluctance to accept reasonable theory until it was proven by sound statistics marked the introduction of each newly discovered blood group system. In this way, dependability and reliability in this new science were universally acknowledged.

The Committee on Medicolegal Problems of the American Medical Association appointed a special Committee on the Medicolegal Application of Blood Grouping Tests. The reports of this Committee were issued in 1952,[30] 1956,[31] 1957,[32] and 1960.[33] The

Committee has not kept pace with this rapidly advancing field, although it has published an increasing list of acceptable blood tests for the guidance of the courts. The Committee also considered the qualifications required of the experts in this new science. These experts were expected to be experienced in the technical aspects of blood grouping tests, well grounded in the principles of inheritance and the laws of genetics, familiar with the production of the various testing serums, and knowledgeable in the endless need for adequate controls.

## Identification of Specimens

The necessity for the correct identification of each blood sample demands a step-by-step, foolproof system. In actual practice this means:

1. Identification of the persons being tested
   a. mutual identification by the involved parties
   b. objective proof of identity: driver's license, auto registration, social security cards, draft board registration
   c. signatures
   d. fingerprinting
   e. group photographs at time of the testing, if possible
2. Identification of specimen in the laboratory
   a. sequential numbering system of original specimen tubes and subsequent test tubes used in the procedures
   b. "double testing"—all tests are done in duplicate by separate technicians working independently. The results are read utilizing "blind" technique (meaning the identity of the specimen is not known to the examiner). All tests are controlled by known testing cells.
   c. comparison of the two sets of findings to insure independent agreement in the results
   d. final classification as to blood groups and conclusions reached by the expert
3. Final report
   a. precise, clear-cut conclusions which would be free of any indecision or doubtful findings or possible misinterpretation

b. a report in language that is comprehensible to the reader, be he judge, jury, or physician.

## ACCEPTABLE BLOOD GROUP SYSTEMS

The report of the Special Committee on the Medicolegal Application of Blood Grouping Tests presented the evidence for the use of the blood group system A-B-O, M-N, and Rh-Hr for medicolegal purposes.[32] To insure dependability, the testing serums approved were those standardized and licensed by the National Institute of Health. However, allowances were made for the use of these other systems by those qualified experts who do have available supplies of the rarer testing serums and the necessary experience in their use. Conclusions reached by such experts using the S-s, Kell-Cellano, Duffy, Kidd, Lutheran and other blood group systems as well as conclusions reached by the use of the inherited characteristics of plasma proteins and erythrocyte isoenzymes may be offered as evidence to the courts. Such exceptionally qualified experts usually prepare their own testing serums and are well versed in their reactions. Unless these reactions are clear cut, the results may not be used in arriving at medicolegal conclusions. As more reliable serums for the newer blood factors become available, the number of blood group systems that can be reliably tested will increase and will be recognized by the courts.

It must be emphasized that blood testing for medicolegal purposes is useful in a negative way; that is, it can be proved that a man is *not* the father of a particular child, or that the blood specimen did *not* come from a certain person, or that a body secretion did *not* come from a given individual. The mathematical chances of proving such exclusions have been calculated by Wiener et al.,[7, 34, 39] Schiff and Boyd,[35] Fischer,[36] Boyd,[37, 38] and others. For example, the chance of proving by blood grouping tests that a falsely accused man is not the father of a given child is shown in Table 1-I.

The formula for calculating the combined percentages for the chance of exclusion using all systems as derived by Wiener[39, 40] is: $P = 1 - (1 - P_1)(1 - P_2)(1 - P_3)$ etc., where P = chance of exclusion in each system. Thus, the chance of exclusion using

TABLE 1-I

| | Single Exclusion Rate % | Combined Exclusion Rate % |
|---|---|---|
| Using the A-B-O system ............ | 20.0 | 20.0 |
| Using the M-N-S-s system ......... | 31.6 | 45.0 |
| Using the Rh-Hr system .......... | 25.0 | 59.0 |
| Using the Kell-Cellano system ....... | 3.8 | 60.0 |
| Using the Duffy system ............. | 7.0 | 63.0 |
| Using the Kidd system ............. | 6.0 | 65.5 |
| Using the Lutheran system ......... | 3.5 | 67.0 |

A-B-O, M-N, Rh-Hr = 51.3 percent and the chance of exclusion using A-B-O, M-N-S, Rh-Hr = 56.4 percent, whereas with the total group listed above, 67 percent of falsely accused men can be excluded.

The additional use of systems such as Kell-Cellano, Lutheran, Duffy, and Kidd can now safely be added to the recommended list of systems since statistical proof of their reliability is at hand. The newer aspects of genetic inheritance, manifested by the study of red cell isoenzymes and plasma protein will still further extend the chance of exclusion. However, the necessity of performing such tests must be limited to those qualified experts whose experience, knowledge, and training preclude the possibility of error.

## GENETICS AND THE LAWS OF HEREDITY
### General Principles

The laws governing the inheritance of the blood groups are derived from the principles of genetics that were first explained by Mendel[41] in 1865. A short review of these principles and their medicolegal application is essential.

Every living organism consists of somatic cells which produce body tissues and germ cells which produce gametes (sperm and ova). In man, the somatic cells contain twenty-three pairs of rods called *chromosomes*.[42] On the chromosomes are located many determinants known as *genes*, each at a specific spot termed a *locus*. Every characteristic of an individual is determined by two genes named *alleles*, these being located at identical loci on each of the paired chromosomes. The *gametes*, however, contain only one member of each pair of chromosomes. In the process of fertilization the two gametes (sperm and ova) meet and combine their respective twenty-three single chromosomes. A complete cell called a *zygote* with its normal complement of twenty-three pairs of chromosomes is formed and a new somatic cell series—thus a new individual—begins.

In this manner, each parent contributes one half of the chromosome pairs which carry the genes that will determine the offspring's individual characteristics. On the pair of chromosomes carrying the genes for the agglutinogens M and N, for example, there must be one gene from each parent to determine this blood type in the child. If the sperm contributes an *M* gene and the ovum contributes an *M* gene, the child's genotype will be *MM*. Such a person having two identical *M* genes is called *homozygous*. On the other hand, if the sperm contributes an *M* gene and the ovum contributes an *N* gene, the child's genotype would be *MN*. Such a person having nonidentical *M-N* genes is called *heterozygous*. Similarly, a person of genotype *NN* having identical *N* genes is homozygous. Thus, an individual can produce gametes (ova and sperm) that carry only one of each of the *M* or *N* genes he possesses. Knowing the M-N types of the parents, it is possible to construct tables of the expected M-N blood types of the offspring of such matings. It is likewise possible to tabulate the M-N blood types of the offspring that could *not* result from each pair of matings.

In the case of the inheritance of the blood groups, the genes determining each of the different blood group systems are located on a different pair of chromosomes. In the independent assortment that takes place, the combinations of the several genes that make up the blood group systems are random in each individual. Thus, the same parents can have children with several different combinations of agglutinogens—*limited, however, to only those agglutinogens and factors present in the parents.*

The laws of independent assortment do not apply to the genes that are located on the same chromosome since each chromosome is inherited as a whole. A rare exception is the occurrence of "cross-over," which has not been observed for the genes determining the blood groups. The genes, which are located on the

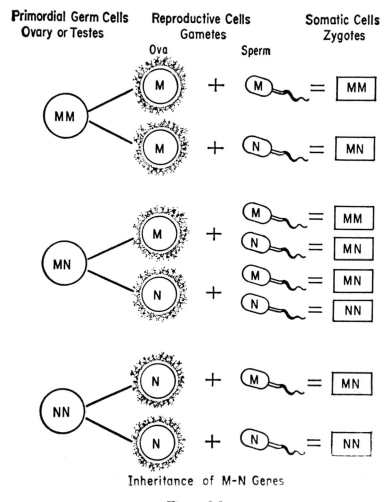

Inheritance of M-N Genes

Figure 1-1

same chromosome but determine different characteristics, tend to be inherited together and create a condition called *linkage.* As an example, the secretor gene and the Lutheran blood group gene have been shown to be linked.[43] The agglutinogens of the different blood groups are determined by multiple alleles each at its specific blood group locus; thus separation or cross-over cannot occur.

## Antigen and Antibody

Almost any blood factor of the red cell agglutinogens can act as an antigen, provoking the production of an anti-antigen (or antibody), when introduced into a person or animal lacking the particular antigen. Anti-**A** antibody is found in the blood of a B person who lacks the A antigen; anti-**B** antibody is found in the blood of an A person. M cells of a human injected into a rabbit results in the production of anti-**M** antibody; similarly, N cells provoke anti-**N**. Antigens vary in their ability to provoke antibodies. Those that stimulate antibody formation easily are called "strong" antigens. Some animals develop antibodies very easily; others are poor antibody producers. It is believed that even the ability to develop antibodies on stimulation is an inherited characteristic. Having available antibody-containing serum, called *antiserum,* for a specific antigen or blood factor permits the identification of this factor on the cells being tested. This is called *cell-typing* and forms the basis of blood grouping tests.

The reaction between a blood factor and an antibody is usually a clearly visible one and results in the clumping of the red blood cells, called *agglutination.* Different conditions may be necessary for this to take place, depending on the particular properties of the antiserum. The reaction may require a saline or a high protein medium. It may take place best at refrigerator temperature ($4°C$), room temperature ($20°C$), or at incubator temperature ($37°C$). Reinforcement of the reaction by special technics such as anti-human globulin, or complement, or enzyme treatment of the red cells may be necessary. Most reactions are time-dependent, requiring incubation for one or two hours to obtain optimal results. The special characteristic of each antiserum must be known to avoid errors, and rigid attention to the details of each technic is essential.

Another type of antigen-antibody reaction is the destruction of the red cell, called *hemolysis.* Complement is needed for this reaction. Since complement rapidly deteriorates on standing, hemolysis is most easily demonstrated when fresh serum samples are tested. Some antigens can only be identified by the hemolytic reactions; others are susceptible to both agglutination and hemolysis.

In the M-N system, there is available both anti-**M** and anti-**N** serums. It is possible, therefore, to test for and identify these blood factors equally. The genes determining these agglutinogens can then be deduced from the tests. In some of the other blood group systems, the necessary antiserums to determine the presence of each of the genes is not available or is not as specific in reaction. Thus, in the A-B-O system it is easy to test for the presence of the A factor by testing with anti-**A** serum. The genotype, however, could be either *AA* or *AO*. To determine this it would be necessary to test with anti-**O** serum which is not available. Since only the A factor can be definitely determined, it is said that the *A* is dominant and the *O* recessive. This terminology is unfortunate since it implies that one gene is stronger than the other. In most cases the genes are equally strong; but some are not as easily demonstrated because the available antiserums are not as avid.

## LAWS OF INHERITANCE

With these brief explanations, the general rules concerning the inheritance of the blood groups can be stated as follows:[44]

1. An agglutinogen cannot appear in the blood of a child unless it is present in *one* or *both* parents.
2. A parent who is homozygous for an agglutinogen must transmit a gene for this agglutinogen to his child.
3. A child who is homozygous for an agglutinogen must have inherited a gene for this agglutinogen from each of his parents.

### Alterations in Blood Type

The value of the blood grouping systems in the study of inheritance results from the complete security that the genes enjoy from any environmental influences. Only in the most unusual and rare circumstances has it been possible to effect any changes in the genes that determine the agglutinogens or in these agglutinogens themselves. A spontaneously occurring accidental modification of a gene is called a *mutation*. Such a phenomena is indeed rare. In man, the frequency of a mutation has been estimated at less than one in 50,000 gene generations.[45] When it does occur, a major disruption takes place which in homozygous form is usually lethal, or causes multiple congenital defects.[46] Acquired changes in an agglutinogen have been reported in the course of severe diseases such as leukemia.[47, 48, 49, 50] These are usually of a partial and temporary nature, and the circumstances of such an occurrence are sufficient to alert the observer. Other environmental toxic influences, such as radiation or chemicals, have no demonstrable effect on the agglutinogens although the mutation rates may be increased.

Some genes can influence other nearby genes and may actually suppress their full expression. This has been reported in the so-called "Bombay" blood.[51] Here, the appearance of the agglutinogen B on the red cell and the B substance in the secretions is suppressed by the actions of the homozygous state of the suppressor gene $xx$. As a factor in causing a seeming contradiction to the laws of inheritance, it is exceedingly rare and easily exposed, since the serum being tested contains anti-**H**, anti-**A**, and anti-**B**.

The only effective way of completely changing the inherited blood type is to replace the entire blood content of the body by exchange transfusion with a different type of blood. This is a therapeutic measure for infants who are affected by hemolytic disease of the newborn (erythroblastosis fetalis). Since the total blood volume of the newborn is very small—approximately one-half pint—an effective replacement can be done with one pint or twice the blood volume. In an adult, whose blood volume is approximately twelve pints, the necessary quantity of blood needed is great and the procedure a formidable one. In addition, the life of the transfused blood is only sixty to one hundred days. Thereafter, the genetically determined original agglutinogens reappear on the newly formed red blood cells. Such temporary alterations in blood type do not pose any serious problems.

Thus, a person's blood typing provides a unique system for identification and for the study of filial relationship. The reliability of the blood type rests on its immutability, since the rare conditions capable of causing any changes are so drastic and unusual as to preclude confusion. The very complexities of the combinations of blood grouping are exactly the quality that makes blood testing so definite and useful in medicolegal work. The qualified expert, supervising the work of careful, dedicated technicians, and following a systematic course of checks and rechecks to avoid technical and clerical error, gives this science the error-free reputation that it warrants.

## OTHER INHERITABLE BLOOD FACTORS

The discovery that the red blood cell was the carrier of inheritable factors that were easily demonstrated in the laboratory, initiated a new era in the study of genetics. The search for individual characteristics was soon rewarded with the finding that the A and B antigens were also present in the saliva and other secretions of 80 percent of all humans.[52] These substances were shown to be identical with the A-B-O type of the person.[53] Individuals could be classified either as secretors or nonsecretors, and the inheritance of this ability to secrete specific substances followed Mendelian laws.

It was also found that some people could distinguish the bitter taste of phenyl-thio-carbamide; others could not.[54] The inheritance of this peculiar character was also shown to follow the genetic rules.

Other elements in the blood were investigated for specific characters of an inherited nature. The leukocytes[55, 56] and the platelets were "typed,"[57, 58] although not nearly as successfully as erythrocytes. The blood proteins next came under scrutiny.[59, 60] Haptoglobins,[61] transferrins,[62] and Gm groups[63, 64, 65] were identified as genetically determined factors. Family studies proved their mode of inheritance. With the introduction of electrophoresis, a spectrum of inherited hemoglobin differences was established. Chapter Six explains further the value and usefulness of the study of these genetically controlled plasma proteins and erythrocyte enzymes as they too follow the laws of inheritance.[66, 67]

To date, these unusual inherited characteristics have not been utilized to any significant degree in parentage studies. The secretor status and the presence of specific genetically determined

A-B-O antigens in the body secretions have been of great value in medicolegal investigations involving the identification of the A-B-O blood types.[30, 68] Differences in haptoglobin types have been used in the Scandinavian countries in paternity cases.[69] This type of evidence is now being presented in the United States Courts. Large numbers of family studies and improved testing serums and techniques for leukocytes and platelet typing and blood protein differences have now been utilized for medicolegal purposes[70] (see Chapter Six).

To further the value of blood group testing in relation to paternity studies, formulae have been devised to estimate the probability of paternity, when blood grouping tests fail to indicate nonpaternity. This subject forms the basis of Chapter Seven by Dr. A. S. Wiener[71, 72] and adds a new facet to this study. Its acceptability in the United States courts will be a matter for future decision.

It is not difficult to see that the increasing number of measurable characteristics that are genetically determined will soon prove that the individuality of a person is his exclusive property, shared only by his identical twin.

## REFERENCES

1. Landsteiner, K.: Zur Kenntnis der antifermentativen, lytischen und agglutinierenden Wirkungen des Blutserums und der Lymphe. *Zbl. Bakt.*, 27:357, 1900.
2. Landsteiner, K.: On agglutination of normal human blood. Translated by Kappus, A. L. from *Wien. Klinische Wochenschrift, 14*:1132, 1901; *Transfusions, 1*:5, 1961.
3. Decastello, A. V., and Sturli, A.: Uber die Isoagglutinine im Serum gesunder und kranker Menschen. *Munchen, med. Wchnschr*, 1090, 1902.
4. Epstein, A. A., and Ottenberg, R.: Simple method of performing serum reactions. *Proc. N.Y. Path. Soc.*, 8:117, 1908.
5. Dungern, E. v., and Hirszfeld, L.: Ueber Vererbung gruppenspezifischer Strukturen des Blutes. *Z. Immun Forsch.*, 6:284, 1910.
6. Bernstein, F.: Ergebnisse einer biostatischen zusammenfassenden Betrachtung uber die erblichen Blutstrukturen des Menschen. *Klin. Wschr.*, 3:1495, 1924.
7. Wiener, A. S.: *Blood Groups and Transfusion.* 3d ed. Springfield, Thomas, 1943. (Reprinted in 1962 by Hafner Publishing Co.)

8. Andresen, P. H.: Reliability of the exclusion of paternity after the MN and ABO systems as elucidated by 20,000 mother-child examinations and its significance to the medico-legal conclusion. *Acta Path. Microbiol. Scand., 24:*545, 1947.

9. Wiener, A. S., Gordon, E. B., and Cohen, L.: Studies on the heredity of the human blood groups. II. The A-B-O groups. *Acta Genet. Med. Gemel., 3:*29, 1954.

10. Landsteiner, K., and Levine, P.: A new agglutinable factor differentiating individual human bloods. *Proc. Soc. Exper. Biol. & Med., N.Y., 24:*600, 1927.

11. Schiff, F.: Die Vererbungsweise der Faktoren M und N von Landsteiner and Levine. *Klin. Wschr., 9:*1956, 1930.

12. Wiener, A. S., and Vaisberg, M.: Heredity of the agglutinogens M and N of Landsteiner and Levine. *J. Immunol., 20:*371, 1931.

13. Landsteiner, K., and Levine, P.: Further observations on individual differences of human blood. *Proc. Soc. Exper. Biol. & Med., N.Y., 24:*941, 1927.

14. Sanger, Ruth: An association between the P and Jay systems of blood groups. *Nature,* London, *176:*1163, 1955.

15. Landsteiner, K., and Wiener, A. S.: An agglutinable factor in human blood recognized by immune sera for rhesus blood. *Proc. Soc. Exper. Biol. & Med., N.Y., 43:*223, 1940.

16. Wiener, A. S., and Peters, H. R.: Hemolytic reactions following transfusions of the homologous group with three cases in which the same agglutinogen was responsible. *Ann. Int. Med., 13:*2306, 1940.

17. Levine, P., Katzin, E. M., and Burnham, L. J.: Isoimmunization in pregnancy, its possible bearing on the etiology of erythroblastosis fetalis. *J.A.M.A., 116:*825, 1941.

18. Levine, P., Burnham, L., Katzin, E. M., and Vogel, P.: The role of isoimmunization in the pathogenesis of erythroblastosis fetalis. *Am. J. Obst. & Gynec., 42:*925, 1941.

19. Levine, P.: The pathogenesis of fetal erythroblastosis. *New York J. Med., 42:*1928, 1942.

20. Walsh, R. J., and Montgomery, C.: A new human isoagglutinin subdividing the MN blood groups. *Nature,* London, *160:*504, 1954.

21. Levine, P., Kuhmichel, A. B., Wigod, M., and Koch, E.: A new blood factor, s, allelic to S. *Proc. Soc. Exper. Biol. & Med., N.Y., 78:*218, 1951.

22. Coombs, R. R. A., Mourant, A. E., and Race, R. R.: *In vivo* isosensitization of red cells in babies with hemolytic disease. *Lancet, 1:*264, 1946.

23. Levine, P., Backer, M., Wigod, M., and Ponder, R.: A new human hereditary blood property (Cellano) present in 99.8% of all bloods. *Science, 109:*464, 1949.

24. Mourant, A. E.: A "new" human blood group antigen of frequent occurrence. *Nature*, London, *158:*237, 1946.
25. Callender, S. T., and Race, R. R.: A serological and genetical study of multiple antibodies formed in response to blood transfusion by a patient with lupus erythematosis diffusus. *Ann. Eugen.*, London, *13:*102, 1946.
26. Cutbush, M., and Mollison, P. L.: The Duffy blood group. *Heredity*, *4:*383, 1950.
27. Allen, F. H., Diamond, L. K., and Niedziela, C.: A new blood group antigen. *Nature*, London, *167:*482, 1951.
28. Layrisse M., Arends, T., and Dominguez Sisco, R.: Nuevo grupo sanguineo encontrado en descendientes de Indios. *Acta Medica Venezolana, 3:* 132, 1955.
29. Sussman, L. N., and Miller, E. B.: Un nouveau facteur sanguin "Vel." *Rev. Hemat.*, *7:*368, 1952.
30. Davidsohn, I., Levine, P., and Wiener, A. S.: Medicolegal application of blood grouping tests. A report of the Committee on Medicolegal Problems of the American Medical Association. *J.A.M.A.*, *149:*699, 1952.
31. Wiener, A. S., Owen, R. D., Stormont, C., and Wexler, I. B.: Medicolegal applications of blood grouping tests. Report of the Committee on Medicolegal Problems of the American Medical Association. *J.A.M.A.*, *161:* 233, 1956.
32. Owen, R. D., Stormont, C., Wexler, I. B., and Wiener, A. S.: Medicolegal application of blood grouping tests. A supplementary report of the Committee on Medicolegal Problems of the American Medical Association. *J.A.M.A.*, *164:*2036, 1957.
33. Sacks, M. S., Unger, L. J. and Wiener, A. S.: Rh-Hr types—Present status. A report of the Committee on Medicolegal Problems of the American Medical Association. *J.A.M.A.*, *172:*1158, 1960.
34. Wiener, A. S., Lederer, M., and Polayes, S. H.: Studies in isohemagglutination. IV—on the chances of proving nonpaternity with special reference to blood groups. *J. Immunol. 19:*259, 1930.
35. Schiff, F., and Boyd, W. C.: *Blood Grouping Technic.* New York, Interscience Publishers, 1942.
36. Fisher, R. A.: Standard calculations for evaluating a blood group system. *Heredity, 5:*95, 1951.
37. Boyd, W. C.: The chances of excluding paternity by the MNS blood group system. *Am. J. Human Genet.*, *7:*199, 1955.
38. Boyd, W. C.: Chances of excluding paternity by the Rh blood group. *Am. J. Human Genet.*, *7:*229, 1955.
39. Wiener, A. S., and Wexler, I. B.: *Heredity of the Blood Groups.* New York and London, Grune & Stratton, 1958.
40. Wiener, A. S.: Application of blood grouping tests in cases of disputed maternity. *J. Forensic Sci.*, *4:*351, 1959.

41. Mendel, G. J.: *Experiments in Plant Hybridization.* (Original in Proc. of Nat. Hist. Soc. of Brunn, 1866) Harvard University Press, 1948. (Translated by Royal Horticulture Soc. of London).

42. A Human Chromosome Study Group: A proposed standard of nomenclature of human mitotic chromosomes. *Am. J. Human Genet.,* 12: 384, 1960.

43. Greenwalt, T. J.: Confirmation of linkage between the Lutheran and secretor genes. *Am. J. Human Genet.,* 13:69, 1961.

44. Sussman, Leon N.: Blood grouping tests—application to related scientific fields. *Am. J. Med. Technology,* 87, March-April, 1965.

45. Neel, J. V.: The study of human mutation rates. *Amer. Nat.,* 86:129, 1952.

46. Haselhorst, G., and Lauer, A.: Uber eine Blutgruppen-Kombination Mutter AB und Kind O. *Ztschr. Konstitutionslehre,* 15:205, 1930.

47. Salmon, C.: Leucémie aiguë et mutations somatique des substances de groupe sanguin. *Rev. Hemat.,* 14:205, 1959.

48. Hoogstraten, B., Rosenfeld, R. E., and Wasserman, L. R.: Changes of ABO blood type in patients with leukemia. *Transfusion,* 1:32, 1961.

49. Tovey, G. H., Lockyer, J. W., and Tierney, R. B. H.: Changes in Rh grouping reactions in a case of leukemia. *Vox Sanguinis,* 6:628, 1961.

50. Ayres, M., Salzano, F. M., and Ludwig, O. K.: Multiple antigenic changes in a case of acute leukemia. *Acta Haematologica,* 37:150, 1967.

51. Levine, P., Robinson, E., Celano, M., Briggs, O. and Falkinburg, L.: Gene interaction resulting in suppression of blood group substance B. *Blood,* 10:1100, 1955.

52. Yamakami, K.: The individuality of semen, with reference to its property of inhibiting specifically isohemagglutination. *J. Immunol.,* 12:185, 1926.

53. Schiff, F., and Sasaki, H.: Der Ausscheidungstypus, ein auf serologischem Wege nachweisbares mendelndes Merkmal. *Klin. Wschr.,* 11:1426, 1932.

54. Blakeslee, A. F.: Genetics of sensory thresholds: taste for phenyl-thiocarbamide. *Proc. Nat. Acad. Sci.,* Washington, 18:120, 1932.

55. Payne, Rose, and Hackel, E.: Inheritance of human leukocyte antigens. *Am. J. Human Genet.,* 13:306, 1961.

56. Gurevitch, J., and Nilken, D.: ABO blood groups in blood platelets. *Nature,* London, 173:356, 1954.

57. Hallgren, H. M., Svardals, J. M., and Yunis, E. J.: Demonstration of A, B and Rh antigens on human leukocytes. *Transfusion (Abstr.),* 6:511, 1966.

58. Pfisterer, H., and Stich, W.: Blood group ABO and Rh in platelet transfusions. *Transfusion (Abstr.),* 6:519, 1966.

59. Smithies, O., and Walker, N. F.: Genetic control of some serum proteins in normal humans. *Nature,* London, *176:*1265, 1955.
60. Harris, H.: Inherited variations of human plasma proteins. *Brit. Med. Bull., 17:*217, 1961.
61. Giblett, Eloise R.: Haptoglobin: a review. *Vox Sanguinis, 6:*513, 1961.
62. Smithies, O., and Connell, G.: Biochemical aspects of the inherited variations in human serum haptoglobins and transferrins. *Ciba Foundation Symposium on the Biochemistry of Human Genetics.* London, Churchill, p. 178, 1959.
63. Smithies, O., and Walker, N.: Genetic control of some proteins in normal humans. *Nature, 176:*1265, 1955.
64. Grubb, R.: Hereditary gammaglobulin groups in man. *Ciba Foundation Symposium on the Biochemistry of Human Genetics.* London, Churchill, p. 264, 1959.
65. Reinskou, T.: Application of the Gc system in 1338 paternity cases. *Vox Sanguinis, 11:*59, 1966.
66. Neel, J. V.: The genetics of human haemoglobin differences: problems and perspectives. *Ann. Human Genet., 21:*1, 1956.
67. Chernoff, A. I.: Some genetic considerations of the abnormal hemoglobins in the light of their amino acid structure. *Am. J. Human Genet., 13:*151, 1961.
68. Wiener, A. S.: Forensic importance of blood grouping. *Exper. Med. & Surg., 2:*44, 1944.
69. Beckman, L., Heiken, A., and Hirschfeld, J.: Frequencies of haptoglobin types in the Swedish population. *Hereditas, 47:*599, 1961.
70. Polesky, H. F.: Paternity Testing, Division of Educational Media Services. *Amer. Soc. of Clin. Path.,* 1975.
71. Wiener, A. S.: Problems and Answers in Immunohematology and Immunogenetics. *Lab. Digest, 38:*8 (Feb.) 1975.
72. Wiener, A. S.: Letters to the Editor: Chances of proving nonpaternity with tests for a sex-linked trait. *Human Genetics,* 1438, 1975.

CHAPTER TWO

# THE A-B-O BLOOD GROUP

BYRON A. MYHRE

## INTRODUCTION

THE DISCOVERY BY Landsteiner in 1901[31] of the existence of in-
traspecies differences in human blood established the presence of what later became known as the A-B-O group system.
Subsequent studies have shown this to be one of the most important blood groups possessed by man.

The A-B-O group is transmitted genetically by a series of co-
dominant alleic genes which occupy one locus on a pair of chromosomes. The three major alleles in this system are known by the
gene symbols of A, B and O. However, a fairly large group of
alleles for subgroups exist. The presence of these genes induce
the comparable antigen[21] to be formed on the red cell membrane.
The O gene is amorphic and does not induce a reactive antigen.
Since the final antigenic structure is determined by the combined action of both genes, the individual may be either *homozygous* or *heterozygous* for a particular blood factor.

The antigens have been studied biochemically[63] and have been
found to be polysaccharides. A and B substances are extremely
stable and have been demonstrated to persist for thousands of
years.[51] They are found in almost all human tissues,[26, 60] although
they are not present in cerebrospinal fluid, lens tissue, cartilage,
and exist weakly, if at all, in hair and nails.

The A-B-O antibodies occur in all healthy individuals and
begin to appear in detectable amounts at about three to six
months of age. The antibodies are directed against the antigens
which are not present on the person's red cells. The titer of the
antibodies usually reaches the maximum at about five to ten
years and begins to decline after that. Most of the antibodies
are IgM immunoglobulins, bind complement, often produce he-

21

molysis when combined with reactive red cells and do not cross the placenta.

## SEROLOGY

### Red Cell Antigens

Division of red cells into A-B-O groups is accomplished by reacting the red cells with anti-**A** serum and anti-**B** grouping serum. Likewise, the serum of the red cells can be tested with known A and B cells ("reverse" or "back-types") to see what antibodies are present. The results of these studies and their interpretations are shown in Table 2-I.

The reaction of red cells with antisera results in the clumping together of red cells into masses which can be seen with the naked eye. This clumping, called *agglutination,* occurs when the antigenic configuration of the red cell is comparable to that of the antibody. The antibody, which has five combining sites (if it is an IgM antibody), reacts with the multiple antigenic sites of the red cell and produces a lattice complex which becomes insoluble and rapidly settles.

A human serum normally does not contain an antibody which will agglutinate its own red cells except in some unusual and usually serious disease states. In the A-B-O system, the serum regularly contains the specific antibody against the absent antigens. Therefore, the A-B-O type of the individual can be determined by:

1. testing the red cells with anti-**A** and anti-**B** serum to determine the antigens present on the red cell and

TABLE 2-I

A-B-O CELL AND SERUM GROUPING

| Genotype | Blood Group Phenotype | Antigens on Red Cell | Antibody in Serum |
|---|---|---|---|
| O/O | O | None | Anti-**A** and Anti-**B** |
| A/A | A | **A** | Anti-**B** |
| A/O | | | |
| B/B | B | **B** | Anti-**A** |
| B/O | | | |
| AB | AB | **AB** | None |

2. confirming the typing of the cell by testing the serum with known A and B cells to determine the antibody or antibodies present in the serum.

The information obtained permits the classification of a person into one of the four major blood groups: O, A, B or AB. These are called *phenotypes* because they "show" the blood type. The genetic composition or *genotype* of the blood type is not as readily apparent since the blood group phenotype is determined by the sum of action of both alleles. Thus, a person with a phenotype of A may be genotypically either *AA* or *AO*. Since the *O* gene cannot be detected, it travels silently and does not influence the phenotype unless it is present homozygously. To determine the genotype of an individual, family studies are usually necessary. For example, when two parents who are blood group A have a child who is O, we know that the genotype of both parents is *AO*.

## Subgroups of A

Blood group A includes several subgroups, the most important being $A_1$ and $A_2$. Anti-A serum produced by Group B and O persons will agglutinate both $A_1$ and $A_2$ cells, but anti-$A_1$ serum will agglutinate only $A_1$ cells. Anti-$A_1$ serum can be made in several ways. It is possible to use serum from B individuals and absorb it with $A_2$ cells so that it contains only anti-$A_1$ activity.[55] This "absorbed B serum" will agglutinate $A_1$ or $A_1B$ red cells but not $A_2$ or $A_2B$ cells. This is only infrequently used at the present time.

The more common grouping method involves using the extract of the seeds of the plant *Dolichos biflorus* which contains a substance that reacts specifically with the $A_1$ antigen,[6, 9] although it apparently does not contain an antibody as it is usually defined. The determination of the $A_2$ antigen allows one to expand the A-B-O phenotypes as shown in Table 2-II from 4 to 6.

Other subgroups of group A have been described and given successive subscript numbers or letters for identification. They are listed as $A_3$, $A_4$, $A_{el}$, $A_m$, and others which are even more unusual. The main importance of the subgroups results from their negative or weak reactions with anti-A serum and from

TABLE 2-II

A-B-O PHENOTYPES AND GENOTYPES WHEN $A_2$ IS INCLUDED
AS AN ANTIGEN

| Phenotypes | Genotypes |
|---|---|
| O | $OO$ |
| $A_1$ | $A^1A^1$, $A^1A^2$, $A^1O$ |
| $A_2$ | $A^2A^2$, $A^2O$ |
| B | $BB$, $BO$ |
| $A_1B$ | $A^1B$ |
| $A_2B$ | $A^2B$ |

the occasional findings of anti-$A_1$ agglutinin in the serum, especially of persons of the subgroups $A_2$, $A_2B$, $A_3$ and $A_3B$. Some of these subgroups of A react weakly or not at all with potent anti-**A** antisera but react with Anti-**A,B** (Group O) serum[70] with a strong or a mixed-field reaction. Other variants of A may not react demonstrably with any antiserum but can be shown to have absorbed the antiserum. All of these subgroups can cause confusion in paternity testing if their existence is not acknowledged, but they are of little clinical significance and can be tested easily in most cases.

## Subgroups of B

There are a few reports of subgroups of B, but these are rare and of little clinical significance.[1, 18, 34, 57, 72] As with the subgroups of A, the subgroups of B are usually detected when anti-**A,B** (Group O) serum is used in conjunction with the other reagents.

## Blood Group Frequencies

In paternity testing it is highly desirable, if not essential, to know the percentage distribution of the various phenotypes in a particular ethnic group so that a rough idea of the number of individuals with a specific phenotype can be estimated. Frequencies in the A-B-O system vary considerably with the race of the propositus. The following gene frequency table, totaled from some much larger and more specific series,[71] will give an idea of this variation (Table 2-III).

The following table should be used for reference only. Any definitive testimony on the various racial distribution of blood

TABLE 2-III*

| Population | O | A₁ | A₂ | B | No. of People in Series |
|------------|---|-----|-----|---|--------------------------|
| White ................... | .67 | .177 | .06 | .093 | 4,845 |
| Black ................... | .685 | .116 | .058 | .141 | 921 |
| Oriental ................ | .605 | .208 | 0 | .187 | 538 |

* Note: This table employs gene frequencies which represent the occurrence of each gene in a random pool of genes taken from the population. To obtain the incidence of a homozygous genotype, the gene frequency should be squared. The incidence of a heterozygous genotype is obtained by multiplying the frequency of one gene by the frequency of the other gene and then doubling this number.

groups should be preceded by studies showing the actual variation in the given population. The variance is sufficient that no specific statements can be made from someone else's study.

## Agglutinins and Hemolysins

Most antibodies of the A-B-O system are IgM immunoglobulins and will bind complement well. If these antibodies are reacted with red cells using fresh serum as a source of complement, the red cells may hemolyze rather than agglutinate. Therefore, any reaction between the red cells and antiserum where hemolysis occurs should be considered a positive test.

The titer of antibodies in a person may vary. The work of Shaw and Stone[50] has shown that antibody titers may vary with the season of the year. This view has been challenged somewhat by Tovey et al.,[62] who could only demonstrate a seasonal variation in individuals from rural areas, but the basic concept of variation has not been challenged. Since some antibodies, especially anti-**B**, may occasionally react weakly and be difficult to determine, this variation should be borne in mind. If serum and red cell groups do not agree, this should be promptly and thoroughly investigated, and the properties should be retested at a later date to see if the antibody strength had been temporarily decreased.

## Secretion

When one is dealing with forensic studies, an integral part of the A-B-O system is the secretor property. The secretor system is determined by two alleles *Se* and *se* which occupy one locus on a pair of chromosomes. The *Se* gene is dominant to the *se*.[48] The resulting genotypes are *SeSe, Sese* and *sese*. The presence of the *Se* gene allows the blood group substances present in the tissue to be acted upon by a series of transferases which cause the substances to become water soluble. The ability to produce a water-soluble substance of A, B and H specificity in the body secretions is present in 80 percent of all humans[32] and is related to the A-B-O blood type. The substances are found in the saliva, sweat, semen, nasal and bronchial secretions, gastric juice, urine, and other tissue fluids. A, B and AB secretors (those possessing the *Se* gene) have specific A or B substance as well as H substance in their body fluids, while group O secretors produce H substance only. H substance is determined by reacting the individual red cells with an extract of the plant *Ulex europaeus*, the common gorse. Since almost all secretors secrete H substance, this test becomes a rapid method for screening of secretion.[8] Saliva from secretors inhibits the agglutination of group O red cells by Ulex anti-**H**; saliva from nonsecretors will not inhibit this agglutination. Testing for the other blood factors can then be carried out in a comparable manner using appropriate antisera. Special care is necessary with $A_1B$ secretors since the H content of these cells is especially weak.

The presence of blood group substance in secretions can be of great value in medicolegal studies. The substance is stable and allows another method of blood grouping when blood stains are not available.

The *Se* gene is inherited independently of the *Le* gene, but does interact with it.[23] Its presence in combination with the *Le* gene causes the red cell to become Le$^a$−, while nonsecretors are Le$^a$+ if they possess the *Le* gene. For a more detailed account, the reader is referred to the work of Watkins.[63] The *Se* gene is found on the same chromosome as the Lutheran blood group gene, and in close proximity to it.[38, 47]

Rare individuals have been reported who secrete H substance but fail to secrete the specific A or B substance expected from their blood grouping. Such persons have been named "aberrant secretors" by McNeil et al.[37] Evidence for subgroup specificity in the secretor substance has also been reported.[57] The careful examination of secretions, properly controlled, can be of inestimable help in medicolegal situations as in examples reported by Wiener.[65]

The human production of anti-**H** is usually confined to those individuals who are of the "Bombay phenotype" which will be discussed later in this chapter. An occasional individual will develop an immune anti-**H**, but their sera are usually so weak that they cannot be used for typing.

## THE A-B-O GROUPING TESTS

Sera for the determination of the A-B-O types are available commercially at relatively low cost. Their reliability is relatively assured since each lot must meet the standards established by the Bureau of Biologics of the Food and Drug Administration as to potency, purity, and safety. This causes the production of an avid, strong antiserum. Since many additives are now introduced into all reagents to increase the speed and strength of reaction, it is essential that the manufacturers' directions for use should be followed carefully. Further, adequate quality control procedures should be established in the laboratory to assure that the reagents are performing as expected and that the results are accurate.

A sample set of directions for use is as follows:

## Cell Typing

**Test Tube Method**

1. Three clean test tubes (10 or 12 × 100) are labeled: anti-**A**, anti-**B** and anti-**A,B** (Group O).
2. Place one drop of the appropriate antiserum in each prelabeled tube. Hold all tubes to the light and visually check for the presence of antiserum in each tube.
3. Add one drop of a 2% to 4% saline (0.9% W/V) suspension of the red cells to be tested. Examine each tube to confirm that red cells have been added.
4. Mix each tube and centrifuge immediately. Disrupt the red cell "button" gently. Examine for the presence of

either hemolysis or agglutination. If none is presented, allow the tubes to remain at room temperature for an additional fifteen minutes. *Do not warm the tubes.* Mix well, centrifuge again and look for hemolysis or agglutination. If neither is present, record the results as negative.

Note: Be sure to run appropriate A and B cell controls simultaneously.

## Slide Method

This method is slightly faster but more subject to error due to drying, rouleaux formation, cold agglutinins and contamination. On the other hand, the slide method is the best method for demonstrating mixed agglutination patterns such as are seen in $A_3$ bloods or in previously transfused individuals.

1. Mark a 1 × 3 inch glass slide in three sections by three vertical lines made with a wax pencil.
2. Place one drop of anti-**A** serum in the first section, anti-**B** serum in the second section, and anti-**A,B** serum in the third section.
3. Add a small drop of the whole blood being tested to each section. The blood should be dropped onto the slide. Take care that the blood dropper is not contaminated by touching any of the reagents.
4. Mix each section with a separate wooden applicator. *Do not heat.*
5. Rotate and tilt the slide for two minutes. Look for the presence of either hemolysis or agglutination which indicates a positive reaction.

Note: The use of anti-**A,B** (group O) serum in A-B-O cell grouping prevents possible errors that can occur if a weak reaction takes place with the anti-**A** or anti-**B** sera. False identification of such bloods as group O is prevented with this method. Also, the antigenically weaker bloods such as $A_3$ or $A_4$ are detected best with this method.

### Serum Grouping

Reverse- or back-grouping is a confirmatory test of the cell typing results. *This test is essential for a valid A-B-O grouping.*

Failure to demonstrate the expected antibody will alert the observer to a possible error in cell typing, weak variants of the red cell antigen, or to the presence of unexpected antibodies in the serum. Serum testing is accomplished best in test tubes.

1. Place two drops of the serum to be tested in each of three tubes labeled $A_1$, B and O.
2. Add two drops of a 2% to 4% saline cell suspension of known $A_1$, B and O cells to the appropriately labeled tube.
3. Mix, centrifuge lightly, or allow to stand at room temperature for one hour. *Do not warm.*
4. Shake gently to dislodge the button of cells and observe for agglutination or hemolysis.

The complete testing system (cell and serum grouping) can be set up at one time in a single test tube rack as follows (Fig. 2-1):
Note: Occasionally the anti-**B** found in the serum of a person who is group **A** will or will not react weakly. The reaction can be strengthened by incubating for twenty minutes at 12°C. If this

| Anti A | Anti B | Anti A,B,(O) | $A_1$ Cells | B Cells | O Cells | Auto |
|--------|--------|--------------|-------------|---------|---------|------|

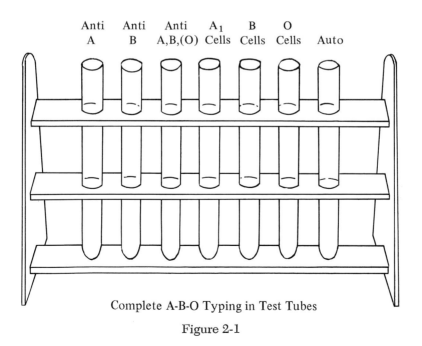

Complete A-B-O Typing in Test Tubes

Figure 2-1

maneuver is used, care should be taken to perform simultaneously an auto control (subject's cells in his own serum) to prove or disprove the presence of cold reacting autoagglutinins.

## Determining Subgroups of A and AB Blood

$A_1$ and $A_2$ subgrouping is usually accomplished by using the plant lectin *Dolichos biflorus,* which is specific for $A_1$ cells. [6, 9] Agglutination identifies the cells as $A_1$.

1. Place one drop of anti-$A_1$ lectin in each of three tubes marked test, $A_1$ and $A_2$.
2. Add one drop of a 2% to 4% saline red cell suspension of the cells to be tested to the first tube, a drop of known $A_1$ cells to the next tube, and a drop of known $A_2$ cells to the third tube.
3. Mix, centrifuge lightly, or allow to stand at *room* temperature for one hour.
4. Disrupt the cell button gently and observe for agglutination.

Positive results are indicated when the test cells agglutinate. The $A_1$ cell controls should agglutinate and the $A_2$ cells should not agglutinate.

## $A_3$

The $A_3$ phenotype occurs rarely but must be considered in any paternity study. It is determined by observing a mixed agglutination pattern when the red cells are reacted with anti-**A** serum or anti-**A,B**. This mixed pattern is best seen using slide grouping technics and is difficult to see with tube methods. The mixed agglutination pattern of very small clumps of agglutinated cells against a field of unagglutinated cells, if seen, should be differentiated by history and supplementary agglutination tests from the blood of a person who just has been transfused and from the blood of individuals who are blood group mosaics or chimeras[17] before one decides the propositus is truly $A_3$.

## $A_4$

The $A_4$ phenotype is found by reacting the red cells to be tested with anti-**A,B**(**O**) serum as well as the usual reagents. No reaction with anti-**A** or anti-**B** and a relatively strong reaction with Anti-**A,B** is indicative of the $A_4$ phenotype. This reaction is probably due to a further blood factor **C** which has been reported by Wiener.[70]

In both the $A_3$ and $A_4$ phenotypes, a significant percentage of the individuals possess anti-**A**$_1$ and the diagnosis can be easily missed if the phenotype is not considered. Fortunately, both types are exceedingly rare, $A_3$ being found about one time in 1,000 individuals, while $A_4$ occurs once in 60,000.[45] Therefore, they will constitute few practical difficulties.

## SECRETOR TYPING

### Secretor Tests

The presence of water-soluble blood group substance in the body secretions can be determined by a screening test using the anti-**H** plant lectin *Ulex europaeus*[15, 16] and anti-**A** and anti-**B** antisera. When body secretions containing blood group substance are mixed with either anti-**A,B** or anti-**H**, the action of the lectin or antiserum is inhibited and they subsequently react less strongly with appropriate red blood cells.

### Screening Test with Ulex Europaeus

The extract of this plant seed which has anti-**H** activity is available commercially. The material to be tested—usually saliva—is obtained as fresh as possible. One milliliter is boiled in a test tube suspended in a water bath for five minutes to inactivate the enzymes present and kill the bacteria. It was found that in large scale studies considerable time can be saved by autoclaving the saliva specimens at 15 PSI pressure for ten minutes. After centrifuging, the supernatant is decanted and used for testing. The lectin or antisera should be diluted before use so that only a 2 plus reaction is obtained against the appropriate test cells. This strength reaction usually requires the dilution of one drop of testing material with ten to twenty drops of saline (final titer about 16). The tests are controlled with known reacting and non-reacting saliva.

a. Place one drop of the diluted lectin in each of three

tubes marked respectively: *test, positive control,* and *negative control.*

b. Add one drop of the prepared unknown secretion, one drop of known positive control secretion, and one drop of negative control secretion to the appropriately marked tubes.

c. Shake and allow to incubate at *room* temperature for ten minutes.

d. Add one drop of 2% to 4% saline suspension of washed group O red blood cells to each of the three tubes.

e. Shake and allow to incubate at *room* temperature for one hour.

f. Centrifuge lightly and read macroscopically.

If the lectin, *Ulex europaeus,* has been inhibited, there will be little or no agglutination of the red blood cells. The saliva, therefore, contains H substance and the donor is a *secretor.* Agglutination of the red cells indicates no inhibition; the donor is a *nonsecretor.* When testing secretions of $A_1$ and $A_1B$ persons, the reactions may be weaker than with the secretions of $A_2$ or $A_2B$ persons. The use of appropriate controls is essential to evaluate these tests.

## Specific Tests with Anti-A and Anti-B Sera

The procedure described above is followed using

    a. Reagents for testing for A substance

        (1) anti-**A** antiserum diluted to produce a 2+ reaction

        (2) saline washed group $A_2$ test cells

        (3) unknown saliva

        (4) known positive A saliva control

        (5) known negative A saliva control

    b. Reagents for testing for B substance

        (1) anti-**B** antiserum diluted to produce a 2+ reaction

        (2) saline washed group B test cells

        (3) unknown saliva

        (4) known positive B saliva control

        (5) known negative B saliva control.

Agglutination in the test tube containing the unknown secretion indicates *nonsecretor* for the specific A or B substance used for the test. The absence of agglutination indicates *secretor* for the substance being assayed in the test. The positive and negative controls must react as anticipated. It is customary to use $A_2$ cells for the A test because of their weaker reactivity which produces greater sensitivity. In testing secretions other than saliva, special technics using varying dilutions of the testing serums must be used.[68]

## PITFALLS IN A-B-O GROUPING TESTS

An almost infallible rule of Landsteiner's states that an adult must have anti-**A** or anti-**B** or both in his plasma if the corresponding antigen is absent in his red cells. Any exception to this rule must be thoroughly investigated. This may necessitate blood group and saliva studies of the propositus and his family.

The conditions in which serum typing may fail to corroborate the cell typing include the following:

### Absence of the Anticipated Antibody
#### Infancy

Transfer of the antibodies through the placenta from mother to child in the absence of active hemolytic disease of the newborn is extremely rare, although possible. Work by Chattoraj et al.,[13] as well as that of others, has established that newborns may make antibodies to the A-B-O blood groups. However, they are so weak that they cannot be used routinely to confirm the red cell type. An infant normally begins to make antibodies in higher levels at about three to six months of age,[39] and his antibody mechanism will be producing almost adult levels at about one year. For this reason, blood groupings on young infants usually have to be done on red cells alone. It is best in these cases to repeat the red cell grouping, preferably using two different technologists and two different antisera, each performing the studies in an independent manner. Care should be taken in these grouping studies to make certain that the child has not had an exchange transfusion or an intrauterine transfusion in the recent past.[59] If so, the reactions are meaningless and could lead to considerable confusion. The tests should be repeated at a later date when the transfused cells are no longer in the child's bloodstream.

## Low Antibody Titer

In elderly or in debilitated persons, the level of antibody may fall.[52] The agglutination reaction may be so weak as to be overlooked. In diseases associated with agammaglobulinemia or in marked hypogammaglobulinemia, little or no antibody may be found. Even a "normal" group $A_1$ individual with no anti-**B** has been reported.[53] Weak reactions can be enhanced by incubation at lower than room temperature; however, the risk of misinterpretation by interfering, cold agglutinins must be prevented by appropriate controls. This is done by the simultaneous testing of several known group O cells with the same serum under the same conditions of temperature and dilution. A further control is that of the "auto" tube—the patient's own cells suspended in his own serum. Agglutination of either of these controls during the test procedure would indicate the presence of either a cold autoagglutinin or of a specific antibody in the serum.

## Chimeras

This rare human occurrence is explained as a result of vascular anastomoses between dizygotic twins. An immune tolerance develops for the blood group antigens of the other twin. The first case reported was a twin of group O whose blood contained some group A red cells. Her serum failed to demonstrate anti-**A** as expected, although normal anti-**B** was present.[17] This extremely rare phenomenon has been reported in several instances[7, 41] and must be considered whenever "defective" groups are encountered.

## Dispermy

In the few cases reported,[40] the serologic findings are similar to those above, i.e. a mixed red cell agglutination pattern. In these cases, however, the propositus apparently begins as one egg fertilized by two sperm and possesses no twin, yet has two genetically inherited blood groups. It too must be considered when considering blood groups.

All of these possibilities need to be considered in any mixed agglutination problem. However, the most common cause of mixed agglutination is a previous transfusion of the propositus,[59] and this should always be considered first.

## Weak Antigens

The subgroups of the A antigen occasionally react weakly with anti-**A** serum. If this weak reaction is not noticed, such bloods might erroneously be classified as B or O; however, the absence of the expected anti-**A** in the serum suggests the presence of a weak antigen. This can be verified by careful retesting with control cells, low temperature incubation, and the use of anti-**A,B** (Group O) antisera. In doubtful cases, the saliva can be studied and elution technics can be utilized on the red cells.[11]

Guy[24] has shown that diabetics occasionally will exhibit weak A-B-O typing reactions. This is apparently due to a water soluble substance present in the patient's serum. To avoid this inhibitor, the red cells should be well washed before use.

The author has seen a similar example in which a patient with carcinoma of the stomach was secreting such large amounts of soluble blood group substance in his serum that anti-**B** typing serum was neutralized before it could react with his group B red cells. This reaction was clarified by extensive washing of the red cells.

The blood sample loses antigenicity as it is stored. Sussman and Butler[58] as well as others, have shown that this loss can be decreased by storing the red cells in an anticoagulant such as ACD which contains a source of glucose as well. Alsever's solution has been found to give comparable results in our laboratory. On the other hand, the blood which is stored clotted will rapidly lose its antigenicity and should be tested as soon as possible.

## Acquired Antigens

Several reports have been published describing an acquired **B** antigen in previously typed group A people. This finding is usually associated with severe disease such as carcinoma[10] or leukemia.[61] The serum typing, however, does not change. The cause of the altered antigenic reactivity has been ascribed to bacterial filtrates,[20, 36] enzymes,[35] bacterial polysaccharides,[54] and possibly to the treatment of the primary disease.[27]

## Presence of Unexpected Antibody

### Agglutination Caused by Drugs

An increasing number of drugs therapeutically administered are cited as causing agglutination of red cells or positive antiglobulin (Coombs) tests. These can cause confusion in both red cell grouping and in the detection of antibodies. Penicillin, cephalosporin, acriflavine,[3] alpha methyl dopa,[73] neomycin among other drugs, have been found to cause this phenomenon. The most common problem in all phases of blood grouping is methyl dopa, which is being prescribed for mild hypertension in an increasingly large number of individuals. This drug can cause erroneous antibody or antigen determinations if the laboratory is not aware of the history of its use. Usually its action is that of a panagglutinin so that one may obtain a suggestion from the serologic studies, but clinical history provides the most aid. Examples have been reported recently of false typing reactions in patients who possess an antibody to caprylate, which is often added as a preservative to albumin.[22] Any albumin-potentiated test should be performed with autocontrols to guard against this mistake.

### Dysglobulinemia

Globulin abnormalities, especially hypergammaglobulinemia, will produce aggregation of the red cells in a characteristic "stack" called rouleaux formation. This can be confused with true agglutination. Differentiation is easily made by examining the clumps under a higher magnification (4-500X) with the microscope (caution—be sure to use a cover slip). If confusion is still present, the aggregates should be mixed with a little saline solution at which time they will easily disperse. Reactions of this type should be considered when the O control cells are agglutinated as well as all the others.

## Cold Agglutinins

Fresh serum of many people may contain cold agglutinins which will agglutinate all red cells, including the patient's own, when the reaction temperature is low. Occasionally the temperature range of these antibodies may be high enough to produce agglutination at room temperature. If the reaction temperature is raised, the aggregates usually disperse. These antibodies are detected occasionally with the current antiglobulin sera which contain significant levels of anticomplement. The reaction is usually weak or inconsistent, and this should serve as a warning as to their presence.

Cold agglutinins with specific activities may belong to the P, Lewis, I, and occasionally M-N systems. Their presence should be differentiated from the cold autoagglutinin by appropriate auto controls and by the identification of the specific antibody.

## Group A Cells with Anti-A in the Serum

The presence of anti-A in the serum when the cell typing appears as A or AB should arouse suspicion that the antigen on the red cell is a subgroup of A, and the antibody has anti-$A_1$ specificity. This finding occurs in 2 percent of $A_2$ and 25 percent of $A_2B$ persons. Subgrouping of the patient's red cells and identification of the specificity of the A antibody will quickly solve this problem.

## Infected Antisera or Red Cells

Gross inaccuracies of cell typing can result from the use of contaminated antisera.[16] For this reason, it is important that the dropper not be contaminated by touching it with hands, glass slides or tubes. The sterility of the contents of the serum bottle must be preserved. Before using the serum, it should be inspected and promptly discarded if not found to be crystal clear.

In like manner, clots of blood used for typing should be tested promptly and stored in the refrigerator in as aseptic manner as possible. Infected red cells have the T sites activated[19] and become panagglutinable.

## "Bombay" Bloods

This type blood, a suppressed variety of the **A** or **B** antigen, was described in 1951 by Bhende[5] and its genetics proposed by Ceppelini[12] and proved by Levine[33] in 1955. These unusual bloods are devoid of A-B-H antigens on their red cells and therefore are usually considered initially as Group O. Subsequent studies will show that unlike O bloods they do not agglutinate with anti-**H** antiserum. Further, their sera possess naturally occurring agglutinins with anti-**A**, anti-**B** and anti-**H** specificities so that they agglutinate all A, B and O cells but do not agglutinate their own red cells. The importance of the "Bombay" phenotype lies in the difficulty of crossmatching these individuals and also in determining the inheritance of the blood groups. The individuals possess a recessive suppressor gene which, when present in the homozygous condition, prevents the A-B-O type from being expressed. However, when this individual has children with a normal mate, the blood group gene is transmitted to the offspring and the now inoperative heterozygous suppressor gene allows the blood type to be expressed. Therefore, the practical situation found would be that two group "O" individuals would conceive a group B (or A) infant. Testing with anti-**H** serum and group O red cells would show that one of the parents was H negative and had anti-**H**, thus being a "Bombay" type. All paternal exclusions of this type should be checked for the presence of "Bombay" type before final reporting.

## Apparent Exclusion Due to Group O Parent Conceiving an AB Child

An unusual family has been reported by Segfried et al.[49] in which an $A_2B$ daughter of an O mother married an O husband and gave birth to two $A_2B$ children. Several other examples are cited by Race and Sanger.[46] In this case the supposition is that by crossing over, both the *A* and *B* genes were duplicated on the same chromosome and that the AB complex thus is inherited effectively as one gene. The extreme rarity of these cases is self-evident. However, they need to be considered in any A-B-O exclusion. Further, one should note that most had a weak ($A_2$)

antigen and that the B antigen also reacts somewhat less strongly than usual.

## MEDICOLEGAL APPLICATIONS

The A-B-O blood group has been of great value in forensic science. Its most frequent use is in matters related to nonpaternity,[56, 67] although its application in solving "mixed baby" and kidnapping cases has been very important. It has also found great use in determining the blood group of blood stains. The genetic laws governing inheritance of the A-B-O blood group are illustrated in Table 2-IV.

The Laws of Inheritance of the A-B-O Blood Group may be stated as follows:

1. Antigens cannot occur in the child if they are not present in the parent.

Example: A group O mother and father cannot have a group A or B child. On the other hand, a group A mother and father can have a group O child since the O gene is an amorph and could be present in the parent's genes without being detected.

2. Antigens cannot be absent in the child if they are present in the parents and should be transmitted.

Example: A group AB parent cannot have a child who is group O. On the other hand, a group A and group O parent can

TABLE 2-IV

A-B-O MATINGS

| Blood Group of Parents | Possible Blood Group of Children | Not Possible Blood Group of Children |
|---|---|---|
| O X O | O | A, B, AB |
| O X A | O, A | B, AB |
| A X A | O, A | B, AB |
| O X B | O, B | A, AB |
| B X B | O, B | A, AB |
| A X B | O, A, B, AB | None |
| O X AB | A, B | O, AB |
| A X AB | A, B, AB | O |
| B X AB | A, B, AB | O |
| AB X AB | A, B, AB | O |

have a group O child if the group A parent has the AO genotype and thus possesses an O gene.

Exceptions to these rules have already been discussed.

### Examples

### Exclusion of Parentage—Typical Cases

a. Alleged father   AB
        mother O
        child     O

Paternity is excluded since an AB parent must contribute either an *A* or a *B* gene to the child. Since the child lacks either A or B antigen, paternity is excluded.

b. Alleged father   A
        mother O
        child     AB

In this case maternity is excluded. The father could contribute the A antigen, or another father could contribute a B, but the mother could not bear a child who is AB. Normally, it is taken for granted that maternity is established and that all exclusions pertain to paternity. However, in rare situations, there may be questions as to maternity.

### Kidnapped Child

In such cases, the usual history is that the alleged mother claims to have given birth to the child at home and has no official birth record. Comparable situations may arise over the possibility of hospital exchange of the children. If the mother alone is to be tested, the chances of exclusion are about the same as in a suspected paternity case. If, however, she also names a putative father to the child, the chances of exclusion become quite good since there are more chances for exclusion of the pair than of just one individual.

### Blood Stain Analysis

The examination of fresh blood stains, while still wet, is easily accomplished. Frequently, a seemingly dry stain or blood clot can be teased sufficiently to obtain intact red cells which can be used for the ordinary grouping procedures. Removal of the cells can be aided by adding a few drops of saline to the stain and flushing the saline through the stain by manual agitation or by squirting with a rubber bulb or dropper. The saline suspension is transferred to a small test tube and centrifuged. The red cells are then reconstituted to a 2% concentration and tested as usual.

Analysis of older blood stains can be performed by several methods, but the usual one used, if sufficient stain is present, is the inhibition technic. It is shown schematically in Figure 2-2. The material to be tested should either be scraped or dislodged by repeated washings in saline and transferred into a test tube using a minimal amount of saline. Antisera to be used (usually anti-**A**, anti-**B** and anti-**H**) are serially diluted and dispensed into two sets of test tubes. To each tube in one series is added an aliquot of the saline suspension of the stain, and to the other set of dilutions an equal volume of saline with no stain. A 2% saline suspension of reactive red cells is added to each tube and the end point of agglutination is determined. If the saline extract is found to neutralize several more dilutions of antiserum than the saline control, it may be determined that the extract contained

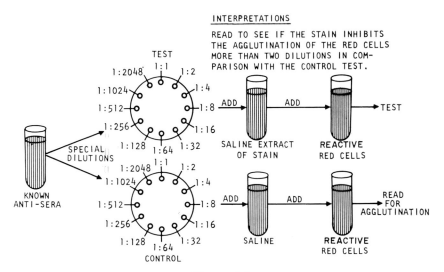

Figure 2-2

this antigen. Currently, the dilutions are usually performed using the microtiter technic.[64] This technic, although quite reliable, should not be attempted without adequate controls and without considerable experience on the part of the person performing the tests.

Analysis of relatively fresh blood stains in small amounts can be performed using other technics which are more sensitive but are technically more difficult to perform.

The absorption-elution technic was introduced by Kind[29] in 1960 and has been extensively modified since then to make the technic simpler and more reproducible. It has been automated recently by Pereira.[43] The simplified method reported by Howard and Martin[28] is the most practical. The usual method used is shown schematically in Figure 2-3. Blood stained threads are teased from the fabric and are placed in boiling McIllvaine's buffer for thirty seconds. They are then immersed in a appropriate antiserum and allowed to remain for two hours. The fiber is washed in saline and transferred to a well slide. A drop of the appropriate reactive red cells is added to each slide and the slide incubated at 50°C for fifteen minutes. If any antiserum has attached to the fiber because of the blood stain antigens, the antiserum will be eluted at the higher temperature and will agglutinate the red cells found in the vicinity. The reader interested in using this technic should consult Culliford's text[15] for the details of the test and practice with known samples for a considerable period of time to gain familiarity with it.

Another technic which has the advantage of working with extremely minute amounts of sample is the mixed agglutination procedure[14] which is shown schematically in Figure 2-4. In this technic the blood stain is treated with the appropriate antiserum,

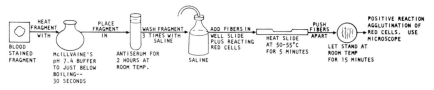

Figure 2-3

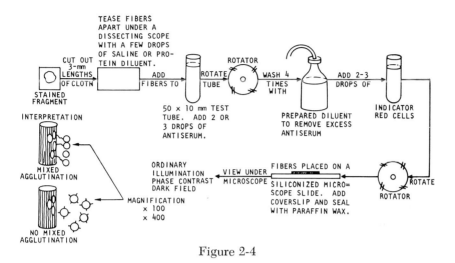

Figure 2-4

washed and immersed in a saline suspension of reactive red cells. The fibers are examined microscopically. A positive reaction is seen when the red cells adhere firmly to the cloth fiber. Again the technical details of this test are important, and it should never be used until considerable experience has been obtained with identifying known blood stains.

### Analysis of Secretions

An interesting case report utilizing the inhibition technic for typing secretions was reported by Wiener.[69] Saline extracts of stains on handkerchiefs used to strangle a victim were found to inhibit anti-**B** serum, which indicated the stains were from a group B secretor. The victim was group A; the suspected murderer was found to be group B and a secretor. The suspect admitted the crime when presented with the evidence.

### SUMMARY

The A-B-O blood group, the oldest system in blood grouping, still remains the one most frequently used in medicolegal work despite its numerous variants and subgroups. In fact, some of its subgroups have increased the usefulness of the group. Its value in paternity testing, personal identification, grouping of old blood stains, and identification of the A-B-O group of secretors makes it a system of great importance in forensic science. Quality control of the antiserum, red cells, and reactions used in A-B-O grouping is necessary to insure reliable and reproducible results. Controls are absolutely necessary to assure reliability of the tests. Finally, a knowledge of the systems, genetics, and the pitfalls which may be encountered is needed to insure accurate interpretation of the results.

## REFERENCES

1. Alter, A. A., and Rosenfield, R. E.: $B_x$ a subtype of B. *Blood,* 23:600, 1964.
2. Alter, A. A., and Rosenfield, R. E.: The nature of some subtypes of A. *Blood,* 23:605, 1964.
3. Beattie, K. M., and Zuelzer, W. W.: A serum factor reacting with acriflavin causing an error in ABO cell grouping. *Transfusion,* 8:254, 1968.
4. Bhatia, H. M., and Solomon, J. M.: Further observations on $A_m^h$ and $O_m^h$ phenotypes. *Vox Sang.,* 12:456, 1967.
5. Bhende, Y. M., Deshpande, C. K., Bhatia, H. M., Sanger, R., Race, R. R., Morgan, W. T. J., and Watkins, W. M.: A "new" blood group character related to the ABO system. *Lancet,* 1:903, 1952.
6. Bird, G. W. G.: Relationship of the blood subgroups $A_1$, $A_2$, and $A_1B$, $A_2B$ to haemagglutinins present in the seeds of *Dolichos biflorus*. *Nature,* London, 170:674, 1952.
7. Booth, P. B., Plaut, G., James, J. D., Ikin, E. W., Moores, P., Sanger, R., and Race, R. R.: Blood chimerism in a pair of twins. *Brit. Med. J.,* 1:1456, 1957.
8. Boyd, W. C., and Shapleigh, E.: Separation of individuals of any blood group into secretors and non-secretors by use of a plant agglutinin (lectin). *Blood,* 9:1195, 1954.
9. Boyd, W. C., and Shapleigh, B. S.: Diagnosis of subgroups of blood groups A and AB by the use of plant agglutinins (Lectins). *J. Lab. & Clin. Med.,* 44:235, 1954.
10. Cameron, C., Graham, F., Dunsford, I., Sickles, G., MacPherson, C. R., Cahan, A., Sanger, R., and Race, R. A.: Acquisition of a B-like antigen by red blood cells. *Brit. Med. J.,* 2:29, 1959.
11. *Committee on Technical Manual: Technical Methods and Procedures.* 6th ed. Chicago, American Association of Blood Banks, 1974, p. 47.
12. Ceppellini, R., Nasso, S., and Tecilazich, F.: *La malattia Emolitica del Neonato.* Milan, Institute Sieroteropico Milanese Serafino Belfanti Milano, 1952, p. 204.
13. Chattoraj, A., Gilbert, R., and Josephson, A. N.: Serological demon-

stration of fetal production of blood group isoantibodies. *Vox Sang.,* *14:*289, 1968.

14. Coombs, R. R. A., and Dodd, B.: Possible application of the principle of mixed agglutination in the identification of blood stains. *Med. Sci. Law., 1:*357, 1961.

15. Culliford, B. J.: *The Examination and Typing of Blood Stains in the Crime Laboratory.* Washington, D. C., U. S. Govt. Printing House, 1971. Stock Number 2700-0083.

16. Davidsohn, I., and Toharsky, B.: The production of bacteriogenic hemagglutination. *J. Infect. Dis., 67:*25, 1940.

17. Dunsford, I., Bowley, C. C., Hutchison, A. M., Thompson, J. S., Sanger, R., and Race, R. R.: A human blood group chimera. *Brit. Med. J., 2:*81, 1953.

18. Dunsford, I., Stacey, S. M., and Yokoyama, M.: A new variety of the human blood group B. *Nature,* London, *178:*1167, 1956.

19. Freidenreich, J.: *The Thomsen Hemagglutination Phenomenon.* Copenhagen, Levin and Murksgaard, 1930.

20. Garraty, G., Willbanks, E., and Petz, L. D.: An acquired B antigen associated with Proteus vulgaris infection. *Vox Sang., 21:*45, 1971.

21. Ginsburg, V.: Enzymatic basis for blood groups in man. *Adv. in Enzymology, 36:*131, 1972.

22. Golde, D. W., McGinniss, M. G., and Holland, P. V.: Serum agglutinins to commercially prepared albumin. *Am. J. Clin. Path., 55:*655, 1971.

23. Grubb, R.: Observations on the human group system Lewis. *Acta Path. Microbiol. Scand., 28:*61, 1951.

24. Guy, R. L., Haberman, S., Romick, I., and Felts, M. H.: Comparison of immune and naturally-occurring antibodies as test reagents for blood grouping diabetic patients. *Transfusion, 1:*138, 1967.

25. Halvorsen, K., and Nordhagen, R.: A modified method of determining the ABO group of blood stains on textiles. *Vox Sang., 12:*312, 1967.

26. Holoborow, E. J.: The distribution of the blood group antigen in human tissues. *Brit. J. Exp. Path., 41:*430, 1960.

27. Hoogstraten, B., Rosenfield, R. E., and Wasserman, L. R.: Changes in ABO blood type in patients with leukemia. *Transfusion, 1:*32, 1961.

28. Howard, H. D., and Martin, P. D.: An improved method for ABO and MN grouping of dried blood stains using cellulose acetate sheets. *J. Forensic Sci., 9:*28, 1969.

29. Kind, S. S.: Absorption-elution grouping of dried blood stains on fabrics. *Nature,* London, *187:*789, 1960.

30. Kitahama, M., Yamaguchi, H., Okubo, Y., and Hazama, E.: An apparently new $B_h$-like human blood type. *Vox Sang., 12:*354, 1967.

31. Landsteiner, K.: Über Agglutinationserscheinungen normalen menschlichen Blutes. *Wein. Klin. Wschr., 14:*1132, 1901.

32. Lehrs, H.: Uber gruppenspezifische Eigenshaften des menslichen Speichels. *Z. Immun. Forsch., 66*:175, 1930.
33. Levine, P., Robinson, E., Celano, M., Briggs, O., and Falkinburg, L.: Gene interaction resulting in suppression of blood group substance B. *Blood, 10*:1100, 1955.
34. Mäkelä, O., and Mäkelä, P.: A weak B containing anti-B. *Ann. Med. Exper. Fenn., 33*:33, 1955.
35. Marsh, W. L., Jenkins, W. J., and Walther, W. W.: Pseudo-B: an acquired group antigen. *Brit. Med. J., 2*:63, 1959.
36. Marsh, W. L.: The pseudo B antigen. A study of its development. *Vox Sang., 5*:387, 1960.
37. McNeil, C., Trentelman, E. F., Kreutzer, V. O., and Fullmer, C. D.: Aberrant secretion of salivary A, B, and H group substances in human beings. *Am. J. Clin. Path., 28*:145, 1957.
38. Mohr, J.: *A Study of Linkage in Man.* Copenhagen, E. Munskgaard, 1954.
39. Mollison, P. L.: *Blood Transfusion in Clinical Medicine.* Springfield, Thomas, 1951, p. 151.
40. Myhre, B. A., Meyer, T., Opitz, J. M., Race, R. R., Sanger, R., and Greenwalt, T. J.: Populations of erythrocytes associated with XX-XY Mosaicism. *Transfusion, 5*:501, 1965.
41. Nicholas, J. W., Jenkins, W. J., and Marsh, W. L.: Human blood chimeras. A study of surviving twins. *Brit. Med. J., 1*:1458, 1957.
42. Nordhagen, R.: Possible sources of error in the blood grouping of dried blood stains on textiles. *Vox Sang., 12*:315, 1967.
43. Pereira, M.: Cited in Culliford, reference 15.
44. Pretshold, H. B.: Screening salivas of group A subjects for secretors status with anti-A$_1$ lectin *Dolichos biflorus. Am. J. Med. Tech., 32*:277, 1966.
45. Prokop, O., and Uhlenbruck, G.: *Human Blood and Serum Groups.* Wiley Interscience, New York, 1969, p. 32.
46. Race, R. R., and Sanger, R.: *Blood Groups in Man.* Springfield, Thomas, 1950, p. 163.
47. Sanger, R., and Race, R. R.: The Lutheran-secretor linkage in man: Support for Mohr's findings. *Heredity, 12*:513, 1958.
48. Schiff, F., and Sasaki, H.: Der Ausscheidungstypus, ein auf serologischem Wege nachweisbares mendelndes. *Markmal. Klin. Wschr., 11*:1426, 1932.
49. Segfried, H., Wolewska, I., and Werblinska, B.: Unusual inheritance of ABO group in a family with weak B antigens. *Vox Sang., 9*:268, 1964.
50. Shaw, D. H., and Stone, W. H.: *Seasonal Variation of Naturally Oc-*

*curring Iso-Antibodies in Man.* Trans. VI. Congr. Europe Soc. of Haematol. 1957, p. 724.

51. Smith, M.: Blood groups of the ancient dead. *Science, 131:*699, 1960.
52. Somers, H., and Kuhns, W. J.: Blood group antibodies in old age. *Proc. Soc. Exp. Biol. and Med., 141:*1104, 1972.
53. Springer, G. F., and Tegtmeyer, H.: Absence of B antibody in a blood group A₁ person. *Vox Sang., 26:*247, 1974.
54. Stratton, F., and Renton, P. H.: Acquisition of B-like antigen. *Brit. Med. J., 2:*244, 1959.
55. Sussman, L. N., and Pretshold, H. B.: Preparation of Anti-**A**₁ (absorbed-B) serum. *Am. J. Clin. Path., 25:*718, 1955.
56. Sussman, L.: Blood grouping tests in disputed paternity proceedings and filial relationships. *J. Forensic Sci., 1:*25, 1956.
57. Sussman, L. N., Pretshold, H., and Lacher, M. J.: A second example of blood group B₃. *Blood, 16:*1788, 1960.
58. Sussman, L. N., and Butler, J.: Antigen reactivity in pilot tube blood specimens: Clotted blood vs. blood stored in acid-citrate-dextrose. *Transfusion, 4:*195, 1964.
59. Sussman, L. N., and Solomon, R.: Another pitfall in blood group testing for nonpaternity. *Transfusion, 13:*231, 1973.
60. Szulman, A.: The histological distribution of blood group substances A and B in man. *Brit. J. Exp. Med., 111:*785, 1960.
61. Tovey, G. H.: *Changes in the Group A Antigen in Leukaemia.* Proc. VIIth Cong. Europ. Soc. Hemat., London, 1959, p. 1167.
62. Tovey, L. A. D., Taverner, J. M., and Longster, G. H.: The effect of environment on ABO antibodies. *Vox Sang., 19:*64, 1970.
63. Watkins, W. M.: *Glycoproteins.* A. Gottschalk, (ed.). London, New York, Elsevier, 1966, p. 462.
64. Wegmann, T. G., and Smithies, O.: A simple hemagglutinating system requiring small amounts of red cells and antibodies. *Transfusion, 6:*67, 1966.
65. Wiener, A. S.: Forensic importance of blood grouping. *Exper. Med. and Surg., 2:*44, 1944.
66. Wiener, A. S.: The value of anti-H reagents *(Ulex europaeus)* for grouping of dried blood stains. *J. Forensic Sci., 3:*493, 1958.
67. Wiener, A. S.: Application of blood grouping tests in cases of disputed maternity. *J. Forensic Sci., 4:*351, 1959.
68. Wiener, A. S.: *Blood Groups and Transfusion.* 3d ed. New York, Hafner Publishing Company, 1962, p. 278.
69. Wiener, A. S.: Cases from the files of the serological laboratory of the Office of the Chief Medical Examiner of New York City. *J. Forensic Med.* (S. Africa), 9:*127, 1962.

70. Wiener, A. S., and Ward, F. A.: The serologic specificity (blood factor) C of the A-B-O blood groups. *Amer. J. Clin. Path., 46*:27, 1966.
71. Wiener, A. S.: Problems and pitfalls in blood grouping tests for non-parentage. *Am. J. Clin. Path., 51*:9, 1969.
72. Wiener, A. S., and Cioffi, A. F.: A Group B analogue of Subgroup $A_3$. *Am. J. Clin. Path., 58*:693, 1972.
73. Worlledge, S. M., Carstairs, K. C., and Dacie, J. V.: Autoimmune hemolytic anaemia associated with a-methyldopa therapy. *Lancet, 2*:135, 1966.

# CHAPTER THREE

# THE M-N-S-s BLOOD GROUP SYSTEM

ANGELYN A. KONUGRES

## SEROLOGY

THE M-N SYSTEM was the second blood group system to be discovered and is one of the most, if not *the* most, informative of all the blood group systems. In the search for antibodies other than those of the A-B-O system that could distinguish between human bloods, Landsteiner and Levine[1] injected rabbits with human red blood cells. This resulted in the production of two distinctly different antiserums, anti-**M** and anti-**N** (defining the M and N antigens respectively), which divided all human bloods into three types, M, N, and M-N. The two alleles M and N determine the presence of the corresponding antigen on the red blood cells; the three genotypes and the corresponding phenotypes are shown in Table 3-I.

## INHERITANCE OF M-N BLOOD GROUPS

The red blood cell agglutinogens M and N are inherited in each generation very strictly according to the laws of Mendel.[2] Both **M** and **N** are inherited as dominant characters, in that whenever a person inherits either or both antigens, they are present and may be tested for in the individual. They are controlled by

TABLE 3-I

M-N GENOTYPES

| Phenotype | Anti-M | Anti-N | Genotype |
|-----------|:------:|:------:|:--------:|
| M ..................... | + | − | MM |
| N ..................... | − | + | NN |
| MN ..................... | + | + | MN |

two alleles and according to the laws of heredity only two forms may be present in an individual, one inherited from the father and one inherited from the mother.

Because M and N types of red blood cells are inherited in a very strict fashion, Table 3-II can be constructed to tabulate all possible combinations of mother and putative father together with the types of children possible or impossible for them to produce.

The established laws of inheritance governed by basic genetic principles, used at present in disputed paternity, as applied to the M-N types are:[3]

    1. The child may not possess a blood factor which is not present in one or both parents (exclusion of the first order): The agglutinogen M or N cannot appear in the blood of a child unless it is present in the blood of one or both parents.

    2. A child must possess those antigens that the putative father would contribute to his offspring, i.e. a child must not lack a factor which the father must pass on (exclusion of the second order). A parent of type M cannot have a child of type N; a parent of type N cannot have a child of type M. Consideration in the interpretation of exclusion in disputed paternity, on the second principle in the M-N system will be discussed later.

This seemingly simple system has greatly expanded and at present there are over thirty different antigens in the M-N sys-

TABLE 3-II

INHERITANCE OF M-N TYPES

| Parents | Possible Combinations | Impossible Combinations |
|---|---|---|
| M X M | M | N, MN |
| M X MN | M, MN | N |
| M X N | MN | M, N |
| N X N | N | M, MN |
| N X MN | N, MN | M |
| MN X MN | M, N, MN | None |

tem.[4, 5] Many of them are rare antigens; some can be attributed to alleles of M and N and some can not, but are obviously determined by genes which are part of the M-N system. The most important being the S and s[6, 7, 8] antigens.

## FURTHER EXPANSION OF THE M-N SYSTEM BY THE ALLELES S AND s

The two antiserums anti-S and anti-s define the S and the s antigens respectively. The M-N and S-s antigens are pairs of alleles apparently derived from closely linked genes. Any combination of M or N with S or s is possible, and each combination is transmitted unvaried from generation to generation. The linkage between M-N and S-s is believed to be so close as to make these genes inseparable. The rules governing their inheritance permit the enlargement of the M-N system from a simple three phenotype and genotype grouping to one of six phenotypes and ten genotypes. Thus, by including the test with Anti-S and anti-s serum, the efficiency of the M-N system is increased for medicolegal purposes. The *M-N, S-s* genotypes are given in Table 3-III.

Table 3-IV tabulates the possible combinations of mother and putative father and the types of children possible or impossible for them to produce.

The established laws of inheritance used at present in disputed paternity as applied to the S-s types are as follows:

1. The child may not possess a blood factor which is not

TABLE 3-III

M-N-S-s GENOTYPES

| Phenotype | Anti-M | Anti-N | Anti-S | Anti-s | Genotype |
|---|---|---|---|---|---|
| MSs | + | − | + | + | *MSMs* |
| Ms | + | − | − | + | *MsMs* |
| MS | + | − | + | − | *MSMS* |
| NSs | − | + | + | + | *NSNs* |
| Ns | − | + | − | + | *NsNs* |
| NS | − | + | + | − | *NSNS* |
| MNSs | + | + | + | + | *MSNs, MsNS* |
| MNs | + | + | − | + | *MsNs* |
| MNS | + | + | + | − | *MSNS* |

## TABLE 3-IV
### RESULTS OF POSSIBLE M-N-S-s MATING

| Mating | Possible Combinations | Impossible Combinations |
|---|---|---|
| MS X MS | MS | MSs, Ms, MNS, MNSs, MNs, NS, NSs, Ns |
| MS X Ms | MSs | Ms, MS, MNS, MNSs, MNs, NS, NSs, Ns |
| MS X MSs | MS, MSs | Ms, MNS, MNSs, MNs, NS, NSs, Ns |
| MSs X MSs | MS, Ms, MSs | MNS, MNSs, MNs, NS, NSs, Ns |
| MSs X Ms | Ms, MSs | Ms, MNS, MNSs, MNs, NS, NSs, Ns |
| Ms X Ms | Ms | MS, MSs, MNS, MNSs, MNs, NS, NSs, Ns |
| MS X NS | MNS | MS, MSs, Ms, MNSs, MNs, NS, NSs, Ns |
| MS X Ns | MNSs | MS, MSs, Ms, MNS, MNs, NS, NSs, Ns |
| MS X NSs | MNS, MNSs | MS, MSs, Ms, MNs, NS, NSs, Ns |
| MSs X NSs | MNSs, MNS, MNs | MS, MSs, Ms, NS, NSs, Ns |
| MSs X Ns | MNSs, MNs | MS, MSs, Ms, MNS, NS, NSs, Ns |
| Ms X Ns | MNs | MS, MSs, Ms, MNS, MNSs, NS, NSs, Ns |
| NS X NS | NS | MS, MSs, Ms, MNS, MNSs, MNs, NSs, Ns |
| NS X Ns | NSs | MS, MSs, Ms, MNS, MNSs, MNs, NS, Ns |
| NS X NSs | NS, NSs | MS, MSs, Ms, MNS, MNSs, MNs, Ns |
| NSs X NSs | NSs, NS, Ns | MS, MSs, Ms, MNS, MNSs, MNs |
| Ns X NSs | NSs, Ns | MS, MSs, Ms, MNS, MNSs, MNs, NS |
| Ns X Ns | Ns | MS, MSs, Ms, MNS, MNSs, MNs, NS, NSs |
| MNS X MNS | MS, NS, MNS | MSs, Ms, MNSs, MNs, NSs, Ns |
| MNS X MNs | MSs, NSs, MNSs | MS, Ms, MNS, MNs, NS, Ns |
| MNS X MNSs | MSs, MS, NSs, NS, MNSs, MNS | Ms, MNs, Ns |
| MNSs X MNSs | MS, MSs, Ms, MNS, MNSs, MNs, NS, NSs, Ns | None |
| MNSs X MNs | MSs, Ms, MNSs, MNs, NSs, Ns | MS, MNS, NS |
| MNs X MNs | Ms, MNs, Ns | MS, MSs, MNS, MNSs, NS, NSs |

present in one or both parents; the agglutinogen S or s cannot appear in the blood of a child unless it is present in the blood of one or both parents.

2. A child must possess those antigens that the putative father would contribute to his offspring, i.e. a child must not lack a factor which the father must pass on. A parent of type S−s+ cannot have a child of type S+s−; a parent of type S+s− cannot have a child of type S−s+. However, the results have to be interpreted cautiously in this second class of exclusions because of the $S^u$ factor.

## U Factor—$S^u$

The antibody, anti-U, which agglutinates the red cells of all white people, but fails to agglutinate the red cells of twelve out of

TABLE 3-V

S-s GENOTYPES

| Phenotype | Anti-S | Anti-s | Genotype |
|---|---|---|---|
| S ..................... | + | 0 | SS, SS$^u$ |
| Ss .................... | + | + | Ss |
| s ..................... | 0 | + | ss, sS$^u$ |
| S$^u$ .................... | 0 | 0 | S$^u$S$^u$ |

TABLE 3-VI

RESULTS OF POSSIBLE S-s MATING

| Mating | Genotype | Possible Combinations | Impossible Combinations |
|---|---|---|---|
| S X S ...... | SS X SS<br>SS$^u$ X SS$^u$<br>SS X SS$^u$ | SS, SS$^u$, S$^u$S$^u$ | Ss, ss, sS$^u$ |
| S X Ss ..... | SS X Ss<br>SS$^u$ X Ss | SS, Ss, SS$^u$, S$^u$s | ss, S$^u$S$^u$ |
| Ss X Ss .... | Ss X Ss | SS, Ss, ss | SS$^u$, sS$^u$, S$^u$S$^u$ |
| s X s ...... | ss X ss<br>sS$^u$ X sS$^u$<br>ss X sS$^u$ | ss, sS$^u$, S$^u$S$^u$ | SS, SS$^u$, Ss |
| s X S$^u$ ..... | ss X S$^u$S$^u$<br>sS$^u$ X S$^u$S$^u$ | sS$^u$, S$^u$S$^u$ | SS, ss, Ss, SS$^u$ |
| S X S$^u$ ..... | SS X S$^u$S$^u$<br>SS$^u$ X S$^u$S$^u$ | SS$^u$, S$^u$S$^u$ | SS, ss, Ss, sS$^u$ |
| S$^u$ X S$^u$ .... | S$^u$S$^u$ X S$^u$S$^u$ | S$^u$S$^u$ | SS, ss, Ss, SS$^u$, sS$^u$ |

approximately 1,000 blacks, was described in 1953.[9] When the second example of anti-U was found,[10] it was observed that blood not agglutinated by anti-U were also not agglutinated by anti-S or anti-s and that all S−s− blood samples were U−. However, later blood samples showed there were two types of S−s−; those that are S−s−U− (84% of random S−s− Negro blood tested) and S−s−U+ (16% of random S−s− Negro blood tested).[11, 12] The U factor is not simple. There is evidence that it is heterogeneous; however, the symbol $S^u$ and the interpretation of $S^u$ being an allele of Ss is satisfactory. This classification of the phenotypes and genotypes which indicate their inheritance is shown in Table 3-V. The results of possible Ss mating are given in Table 3-VI.

The necessity of caution in interpretation of results obtained in blood tests using both anti-S and anti-s typing serums to determine paternity is shown in the following case:

| RBC | Anti-S | Anti-s | Interpretation Number 1 | Interpretation Number 2 |
|---|---|---|---|---|
| Putative father | + | 0 | SS | $SS^u$ |
| Mother | + | + | Ss | Ss |
| Child | 0 | + | ss | $sS^u$ |

From the test results the putative father appears to be of the type SS and the child S-negative (ss). This would contradict the aforementioned law that a child must possess those factors which the father must pass on. However, he could be of the type $SS^u$ and could father an S-negative child. The two possible interpretations as shown in the above table of this case are: First interpretation, a man who is SS cannot father a child who is ss (paternity exclusion). However, in the second interpretation, a man who is $SS^u$ could be the father of an S-negative ($sS^u$) child (no paternity exclusion). The homozygous (SS) or heterozygous ($SS^u$) status of this man could be determined by additional testing (see dosage test) or possibly by family studies.

### An Additional Example of Paternal Exclusion in the M-N-S-s System

Certain of the blood group antigens are determined by closely linked genes which have been shown to segregate almost always in close association. The possibility of exclusion exists when it can be shown from other children of the same couple how the linked antigens are being passed on. This is not a consideration in most paternity cases, but it does occur in paternity allegations surrounding divorce suits.

This case illustrates an exclusion based on linkage in the M-N-S-s system:

|  | FATHER |  | MOTHER |  |
|---|---|---|---|---|
|  | MNSs |  | MSs |  |
|  | Ms-NS |  | MS-Ms |  |
| CHILDREN | #1 | #2 | #3 | #4 |
|  | MS-NS | MS-NS | MS-Ms | Ms-Ns |

In this mating it can be seen from the first three offspring that so far as the father is concerned, *M* is transmitted packaged with *s*, and *N* with *S*. Therefore, the M-N-S-s group of the fourth child is such that if the putative father is not excluded, another man must be the father of the first three children. The fourth child has Ms which it obviously received from the mother and must then have received Ns from its father. The alleged father in this case, however, could not have contributed Ns and is, therefore, not the actual father.

**Variants**

The M-N-S-s and the phenotype S$^u$ which have been described make up the main skeleton of the M-N-S-s system. There are many other antigens (mostly rare) associated with the M-N-S-s system. The antigens of the M-N-S-s system may be divided into two classifications:

1. Variants that appear to represent alleles at the MN or Ss loci, or both. These are usually detected by their failure to react with some or all of the standard anti-**M**, -**N**, -**S** or anti-**s** serums.
2. Variant antigens that are detected by specific antiserum. These antigens are dominant characters and their genes are closely linked to, or part of, the M-N-S-s complex locus. These antigens are almost always very rare.

In paternity testing only the antigens that appear to represent alleles need be considered. Others are of little medicolegal importance.

## Alleles at the MNSs Locus

### $N_2$

$N_2$,[13, 14] a weak N antigen is weakly agglutinated by most anti-N serums but not agglutinated by others. It is essential that M and N testing be done with two or three different serums. Adequate controls should always be included in all M and N testing.

### $M^g$

$M^g$[15], an extremely rare (1 in 44,000)[16, 17] antigen of the M-N system that does not react with anti-M or anti-N serum, but does react with a specific antibody, anti-$M^g$. Its importance rests in the danger of an erroneous exclusion of parentage where the alleged parent and child are of different MN types. An $M^g$N person will appear as NN when using only anti-M and anti-N. Similarly an $M^g$M individual tests as MM. However, blood representing the genotype $M^gM$ if tested with only anti-M and anti-N gives the reaction of M, but it gives only the single dose reaction when tested against titrations of anti-M serum. Similarly, blood representing $M^gN$ gives only single dose reactions against anti-N.

The necessity of testing all blood in a MN paternity exclusion with anti-$M^g$, in addition to anti-M and anti-N, is shown in the following case:

|        | Anti-M | -N | -$M^g$ | Phenotype | Genotype |
|--------|--------|-----|---------|-----------|----------|
| Father | 0      | +   | +       | N         | $M^gN$   |
| Mother | +      | 0   | 0       | M         | $MM$     |
| Child  | +      | 0   | +       | M         | $M^gM$   |

Thus, an apparent exclusion on the basis of MN typing becomes invalid. There is no contradiction to the laws of theoretical expectancy in these findings. Paternity cannot be excluded. Furthermore, in view of the infrequency of the $M^g$ blood factor (1:44,000)[16] the finding of this rare blood factor in a child and the alleged father suggests a rather strong probability that indeed he is the father.

## M[k]

M[k 18] is a very rare allele producing no M, N, S or s antigen. Anti-M[k] has been produced in rabbits but gives very weak reactions. However, M[k] is very similar to M[g] in that testing blood donors with dosing anti-M and anti-N, the unexpected single doses revealed further examples (5 out of 3,894 donors) of M[k], which were found to react with the weak anti-M[k] serum. Other rare alleles have been described such as M[c 19] and M[v 20] but are of no medicolegal significance because of their extreme rarity.

There are other gene complexes at the MNSs[19] locus which have been described. The presence of any one of them usually results in less M or N antigen being produced. These may be alternative antigens or possibly the results of position effects i.e. the presence of one antigen may seriously interfere with the expression of another antigen. Therefore, any weak or irregular reaction in testing with anti-M,-N,-S and Anti-s should be evaluated with great caution in medicolegal reports before being considered in paternity exclusions.

### Other Facts About the M-N-S-s System

#### Development of the Antigens

The M-N-S-s antigens as well as the U and M[g] antigens are well developed in the newborn and remain unchanged throughout life.[4]

#### Antibodies of the M-N-S-s System

The antibodies anti-M and anti-N are only rarely present in human serum. They are usually produced by injecting rabbits with the appropriate human red cells. Anti-M and anti-N typing reagents can also be prepared from saline extract of seeds; anti-M from the seeds of the plant, *Iberis amara*,[22] anti-N from the seeds of *Vicia graminea*.[23] Anti-S[6, 7] anti-s[8] and anti-U[9,10] are usually of human origin. Anti-s has been produced in rabbits; anti-S has not. Anti-S may be naturally occurring or immune.[24, 25, 26, 27, 28] All examples of anti-s[29, 30] and anti-U[9, 10] have been immune in origin.

**Dosage Effects**

Dosage of anti-**M**, anti-**N**, anti-**S** and anti-s is very common.[31] Dosage effect is the difference in strength of reactivity of an antigen in the homozygous from that in the heterozygous state, and can be tested for by titration methods.[30] These variations in amount (depending on the genetic constitution of the donor) can be recognized and roughly measured by comparing strengths of the reactions when different cell samples are tested against parallel titrations of the antiserum.

Dosage with anti-**M**, -**N**, -**S** and anti-s have been very useful in the understanding of most of the newer alleles of this system, particularly $M^g$ and $M^k$.[21, 33]

**Test for M and N Types**

All MN tests should be done in duplicate, using separate lots of serum by two technics if possible. This testing should always include bloods of known M and N types for controls.

SLIDE TESTS:

1.  A 4% saline suspension of the washed, unknown cells, known M cells, MN cells and N cells is prepared.
2.  A drop of anti-**M** serum is placed in each of the number of wells equal to the number of unknowns plus the wells for the three control cells.
3.  A drop of anti-**N** serum is similarly distributed in another set of wells to include the total number of unknowns plus the three control cells.
4.  A drop of the RBC suspensions is added to the appropriately marked wells and thoroughly mixed.
5.  The slides are either:

    (a) Incubated at room temperature for several minutes— depending on the length of time required for reactions to occur with the positive control while the negative control cells remain evenly suspended, or (b) placed on a mechanical rotator for approximately ten minutes, after which the controls are inspected. If these are satisfactory, the unknown can then be read.

TUBE TEST:

1. A 2% saline suspension of the washed, unknown cells, known M cells, MN cells and N cells is prepared.
2. For each specimen, label two (10 × 75mm) tubes; one "M" and the second "N."
3. Add one drop of anti-**M** to tubes labelled "M."
4. Add one drop of anti-**N** to tubes labelled "N."
5. Add one drop of the 2% saline suspension of cells for each specimen to appropriately labelled tubes.
6. Mix well, allow to stand at room temperature or at 4°C for one hour, depending on the time necessary to produce clean-cut positive and negative reactions in the controls.
7. Examine for agglutination.

   Note: If bloods are to be tested at 4°C, a control for cold agglutination using 5% albumin instead of the specific typing serum is done.

## Test for S and s Types:

The tests are best performed with anti-**S** and anti-**s** serums at 37°C followed by antihuman globulin test. Tests with red cells homozygous and heterozygous for S and s should be included as controls. Furthermore, the manufacturer's procedures when using typing serums and/or antihuman globulin reagents should be followed.

1. For each specimen to be tested, label two (10 × 75mm) tubes; one "S" and the second "s."
2. Into each of the appropriately labelled tubes, place one or two drops (depending on manufacturer's recommendations) of known antisera to be used, i.e. anti-**S** in tube "S"; anti-**s** in tube "s."
3. Into each of the appropriately labelled tubes, place one drop of 2% saline suspension of unknown cells, known positive control cells and known negative control cells and known heterozygous (Ss) blood.
4. Mix well; incubate at 37°C for one hour (incubation time depends on the manufacturer's instructions).

5. Wash three times with normal saline. Decant excess saline after last wash by a quick flip of the wrist.
6. Add one or two drops of antihuman globulin.
7. Mix well; centrifuge one minute at 1,500 rpm.
8. Gently dislodge button. Read for agglutination.

BLOOD TESTING IN THE M-N-S-s SYSTEM MUST ALWAYS INCLUDE CONTROLS OF KNOWN TYPES. AS ALWAYS, SIMULTANEOUS TESTING OF UNKNOWN BLOODS WITH THE SAME SERUMS AND UNDER THE SAME CONDITIONS OF TIME AND TEMPERATURE MUST BE PERFORMED TO AVOID THE POSSIBILITY OF ANY FALSE OBSERVATIONS.

## MEDICOLEGAL CONCLUSIONS

The M-N-S-s system provides a very significant and efficient blood group for parentage studies because of the distinctly demonstrable genes which travel inseparably from parent to child.[34, 35] The calculated probability that a falsely accused man will be excluded by testing for the factors M-N-S-s is 31.58 percent. If only anti-**M** and anti-**N** serum is used, this figure falls to 18.75 percent.[36, 37] Therefore, a falsely accused defendant deserves the benefit of the highest probable exclusion advantage and should be tested with anti-**M**, anti-**N**, anti-**S** and anti-**s** serums.

## REFERENCES

1. Landsteiner, K., and Levine, P.: On individual differences in human blood. *J. Exper. Med., 47*:757, 1928.
2. Landsteiner, K., and Levine, P.: On inheritance of agglutinogens of human blood demonstrable by immune agglutinins. *J. Exper. Med., 48*:731, 1928.
3. Davidsohn, I., Levine, P., and Wiener, A. S.: Medicolegal application of blood grouping tests. A report of the Committee on Medicolegal Problems of the American Medical Association. *J.A.M.A., 149*:699, 1952.
4. Race, R. R., and Sanger, R.: *Blood Groups in Man.* Ed. 1-5, Philadelphia, F. A. Davis, 1950, 1954, 1958, 1962 and 1968.
5. Issitt, P. D.: *Applied Blood Group Serology.* Oxnard, California, Spectra Biologics, 1970.
6. Walsh, R. J., and Montgomery, C. M.: A new human isoagglutinin subdividing the MN blood groups. *Nature,* London, *160*:504, 1947.

7. Sanger, R., and Race, R. R.: Subdivisions of the MN blood groups in man. *Nature*, London, *160:*595, 1947.

8. Levine, P., Kuhmichel, A. B., Wigod, M., and Koch, E.: A new blood factor, s, allelic to S. *Proc. Soc. Exper. Biol. & Med., N. Y., 78:*218, 1951.

9. Wiener, A. S., Unger, L. J., and Gordon, E. B.: Fatal hemolytic transfusion reaction caused by sensitization to a new blood factor U. *J.A.M.A., 153:*1444, 1958.

10. Greenwalt, T. J., Sasaki, T., Sanger, R., Sneath, J., and Race, R. R.: An allele of the S(s) blood group genes. *Proc. Nat. Acad. Sci., 40:*1126, 1954.

11. Allen, F. H., Jr., Madden, Helen J., and King, R. W.: The MN gene MU, which produces M and U but no N, S or s. *Vox Sang., 8:*549-556, 1963.

12. Francis, Betty J., and Hatcher, D. E.: MN blood types. The $S^-s^-U^+$ and the $M_1$ phenotypes. *Vox Sang., 11:*213-216, 1966.

13. Crome, W.: Uber Blutgruppenfragen: Mutter M, Kind N. *Dtsch. Ztschr. gerichtl. Med., 24:*167-175, 1935.

14. Friedenreich, V.: Ein erblicher defekter N-Receptor, der wahrscheinlich eine bisher unbekannte blutgruppeneigenschaft innerhalb des MN-Systems darstellt. *Dtsch Ztschr. gerichtl. Med., 25:*358-368, 1939.

15. Allen, F. H., Corcoran, Patricia A., Kenton, H. B., and Breare, Nancy: $M^g$, a new blood group antigen in the MNS system. *Vox Sang., 3:*81-91, 1958.

16. Winter, N. M., Antonelli, G., Walsh, E. A., and Konugres, A. A.: A second example of blood group antigen $M^g$ in the American population. *Vox Sang., 11:*209-212, 1966.

17. Sussman, L. N., Boruck, D. T., and Pretshold, H.: A study of the gene $M^g$ in a paternity case. *Medical Lab.* December 1961, pp. 28-29.

18. Metaxas, M. N., and Metaxas-Buhler, M.: $M^k$: an apparently silent allele at the MN locus. *Nature*, London, *202:*1123, 1964.

19. Dunsford, I., Iken, Elizabeth W., and Mourant, A. E.: A human blood group gene intermediate between M and N. *Nature*, London, *172:*688-689, 1953.

20. Gershowitz, H., and Fried, K.: Anti-$M^v$, a new antibody of the MNS blood group system. I. $M^v$, a new inherited variant of the M gene. *Amer. J. Human Genet., 18:*264-281, 1966.

21. Metaxas, M. N., Metaxas-Buhler, Margrit, and Ikin, Elizabeth W.: Complexities of the MN Locus. *Vox Sang., 15:*102-117, 1968.

22. Bird, G. W. G.: Observations on some non-specific plant haemagglutinins. *Vox Sang., 4:*318-319, 1959.

23. Ottensooser, F., and Silberschmidt, K.: Haemagglutinin anti-N in plant seeds. *Nature*, London, *172:*914, 1953.

24. Coombs, H. I., Ikin, Elizabeth W., Mourant, A. E., and Plaut, Gertrude: Agglutinin anti-S in human serum. *Brit. Med. J., i:*109-111, 1951.

25. Constantoulis, N. C., Paidoussis, M., and Dunsford, I.: A naturally occurring anti-s agglutinin. *Vox Sang. (O.S.),* 5:143-144, 1955.

26. Pickles, Margaret M.: A further example of the anti-S agglutinin. *Nature,* London, *162:*66, 1948.

27. Levine, P., Ferraro, L. R., and Koch, Elizabeth: Hemolytic disease of the newborn due to anti-S. *Blood,* 7:1030-1037, 1952.

28. Cutbush, Marie, and Mollison, P. L.: Haemolytic transfusion reaction due to anti-S. *Lancet, ii:*102-103, 1949.

29. Sanger, Ruth, Race, R. R., Rosenfield, R. E., and Vogel, P.: A serum containing anti-s and anti-Jk[b]. *Vox Sang. (O.S.),* 3:71, 1953.

30. Fudenberg, H., and Allen, F. H.: The blood group antibody anti-s: a third example. *Vox Sang.,* 2:133-137, 1957.

31. Sanger, Ruth, and Race, R. R.: The MNSs blood group system. *Amer. J. Human Genet.,* 3:332-343, 1951.

32. Sussman, L. N.: Titration and scoring in disputed parentage. *Transfusion,* 5:248-252, 1965.

33. Metaxas-Buhler, M., Cleghorn, T. E., Romanski, J., and Metaxas, M. N.: Studies on the blood group antigen M[g]. II. Serology of M[g]. *Vox Sang.,* 11:170-183, 1966.

34. Wiener, A. S.: *Blood Groups and Transfusion.* 3d edition, Springfield, Thomas, 1943.

35. Sussman, L. N.: *Blood Grouping Tests. Medico-Legal Uses.* Springfield, Thomas, 1968.

36. Wiener, A. S.: Heredity of the M-N-S blood types. Theoreticostatistical considerations. *Amer. J. Human Genet.,* 4:37, 1952.

37. Boyd, W. C.: The chances of excluding paternity by the MNS blood group system. *Amer. J. Human Genet.,* 7:199, 1955.

CHAPTER FOUR

# THE Rh-Hr BLOOD GROUPS

## HISTORICAL DEVELOPMENT

LEON N. SUSSMAN

LANDSTEINER AND WIENER,[1] in 1940, published a paper describing a new human antigen present in 85 percent of Caucasians, which they called Rh. The new antigen was recognized by an antiserum produced in the rabbit following the injection of the blood of the Rhesus monkey, hence the name Rh. Their discovery stimulated a new area of laboratory medicine—immunohematology—and represented a contribution of the utmost importance to blood grouping and transfusion therapy. Aided by the greatly expanded use of blood during World War II, the science of immunohematology blossomed; hundreds of papers on the subject of Rh were published in the next few years.

The relationship of the Rh system to intragroup transfusion reactions[2] and to hemolytic disease of the newborn[3] established the vital clinical significance to the discovery. Geneticists quickly tested the theories concerning the inheritance of the Rh factor with thousands of family studies.[4, 5] In the meanwhile, the laboratory investigators explored the complexities of the new blood group system and worked at solving many of the riddles posed by unusual and unexpected findings. To attempt more than a short summary of the Rh system is beyond the scope of this text. The interested reader is referred to the numerous excellent books on the subject, including those by Wiener,[6, 7] Race and Sanger,[5] Wiener and Wexler,[8] Boorman and Dodd,[9] and Erskine.[10]

### THE RH-HR SUBGROUPS

The originally described rabbit anti-**Rh** serum was shown to detect the presence of only one of several Rh antigens although the most important. This was named **Rh**$_0$ by Wiener, indicating by a capital R its priority and importance, since 90 percent of clinical conditions involving the new blood group system related to $Rh_0$. Other antigens were soon described and given places in the nomenclature based on their time of discovery, their clinical significance, and their relationship to each other. These were successively named **rh'**[11] (present in 70% of Caucasians), and **rh''**[12, 13, 14] (present in 30% of Caucasians). The three antiserums enabled the construction of Table 4-I by Wiener[15] who proposed the accompanying nomenclature.

The finding by Levine[16, 17] of an antiserum which recognized the allele of **rh'**, enabled further differentiation of the phenotype rh' and its probable genotypes. This new antibody was called anti-**hr'** (the opposite of **rh'**). Soon thereafter the allele of **rh''** was found and named **hr''**[18, 19] to correspond to the **rh'-hr'** relationship. The search for the counterpart of $Rh_0$ which would have permitted a more complete classification of the Rh-Hr types was unsuccessful; this served to point up the complex nature and unique position of the $Rh_0$ factor in the system. The additional advantages offered by the use of anti-**hr'** and anti-**hr''** permit the construction of a more complex classification, including the most likely genotype as well as the other possible genotypes (Table 4-II). The most likely genotype is determined by the estimated gene frequency among Caucasians. The "most frequent genotype" and the figures for the frequency of the phenotypes and the genotypes will vary of course with the ethnic group being studied.[20]

To explain the complexities of the Rh-Hr blood group system,

TABLE 4-I

Rh TYPES

|  | anti-$Rh_0$ | anti-rh' | anti-rh'' |
|---|---|---|---|
| rh (neg) | − | − | − |
| rh' | − | + | − |
| rh'' | − | − | + |
| $rh_y$ (rh'rh'') | − | + | + |
| $Rh_0$ | + | − | − |
| $Rh_1$ ($Rh_0'$) | + | + | − |
| $Rh_2$ ($Rh_0''$) | + | − | + |
| $Rh_z$ ($Rh_1Rh_2$) | + | + | + |

## TABLE 4-II

## Rh-Hr PHENOTYPES AND GENOTYPES (CAUCASIANS)

| Phenotype | Rh Antisera $Rh_0$ | rh' | rh'' | Hr Antisera hr' | hr'' | hr | Phenotype | Freq. | Most Freq. Genotype | Freq. | Other Genotypes | |
|---|---|---|---|---|---|---|---|---|---|---|---|---|
| rh | − | − | − | + | + | + | rh | 14.4 | $rr$ | 14.4 | None | |
| rh' | − | + | − | + | + | + | rh'rh | 0.46 | $r'r$ | 0.46 | None | |
|  | − | + | − | − | + | − | rh'rh' | 0.0036 | $r'r'$ | 0.0036 | None | |
| rh'' | − | − | + | + | + | + | rh''rh | 0.38 | $r''r$ | 0.38 | None | |
|  | − | − | + | + | − | − | rh''rh'' | 0.0025 | $r''r''$ | 0.0025 | None | |
| $rh_y$ | − | + | + | + | + | − | rh'rh'' | 0.006 | $r'r''$ | 0.006 | None | |
|  | − | + | + | + | + | + | $rh_y$rh | 0.008 | $r^y r$ | 0.008 | None | |
|  | − | + | + | − | + | − | $rh_y$rh' | 0.0001 | $r^y r'$ | 0.0001 | None | |
|  | − | + | + | + | − | − | $rh_y$rh'' | 0.0001 | $r^y r''$ | 0.0001 | None | |
|  | − | + | + | − | − | − | $rh_y rh_y$ | 0.000001 | $r^y r^y$ | 0.000001 | None | |
| $Rh_0$ | + | − | − | + | + | + | $Rh_0$ | 2.2 | $R^0 r$ | 2.0 | $R^0 R^0$ | |
| $Rh_1$ | + | + | − | + | + | + | $Rh_1$rh | 33.4 | $R^1 r$ | 31.2 | $R^1 R^0$ | $R^0 r'$ |
|  | + | + | − | − | + | − | $Rh_1 Rh_1$ | 17.3 | $R^1 R^1$ | 16.6 | $R^1 r'$ | |
| $Rh_2$ | + | − | + | + | + | + | $Rh_2$rh | 14.6 | $R^2 r$ | 12.2 | $R^2 R^0$ | $R^0 r''$ |
|  | + | − | + | + | − | − | $Rh_2 Rh_2$ | 2.4 | $R^2 R^2$ | 2.0 | $R^2 r''$ | |
| $Rh_z$ | + | + | + | + | + | − | $Rh_1 Rh_2$ | 12.9 | $R^1 R^2$ | 12.3 | $R^1 r''$ | $R^2 r'$ |
|  | + | + | + | + | + | + | $Rh_z$rh | 0.17 | $R^z r$ | 0.15 | $R^z R^0$ | $R^0 r^y$ |
|  | + | + | + | − | + | − | $Rh_z Rh_1$ | 0.17 | $R^z R^1$ | 0.15 | $R^z r'$ | $R^1 r^y$ |
|  | + | + | + | + | − | − | $Rh_z Rh_2$ | 0.07 | $R^z R^2$ | 0.06 | $R^z r''$ | $R^2 r^y$ |
|  | + | + | + | − | − | − | $Rh_z Rh_z$ | 0.0008 | $R^z R^z$ | 0.0008 | $R^z r^y$ | |

two principal competing theories and nomenclatures were advanced. The Wiener concept[21, 22] postulates that the Rh locus on the chromosome is the site of one of many allelic genes (the multiple allele theory), and this gene is transmitted as a single nondivisible unit throughout the generations. This nomenclature, therefore, provides a single symbol for each allele; this allelic gene determines a single unit on the RBC called the *agglutinogen*. The agglutinogen may be characterized by many blood factors, each one being serologically recognizable by its specific antiserum. To clearly indicate these differences the gene or genotype is printed in *italics*, the agglutinogen or phenotype in normal type, while the blood factor (the serological specificity), and its corresponding antibody is printed in **boldface**.

The Fisher-Race hypothesis[23] postulates three closely linked genes (*D* for *Rh₀*, *C* for *rh'*, and *E* for *rh''*). These are assumed to be so closely linked that they can be considered nondivisible. Nevertheless, there is the implied possibility that "crossing-over" could take place or that separate elements of the C-D-E unit could be transmitted—a situation that has never been reported.[24] the confusion that has resulted from the C-D-E concept has led to laboratory errors in typing and in paternity conclusions. A third

TABLE 4-III

CONVERSION TABLE—Rh-Hr AND C-D-E

| Wiener | Fisher-Race |
|---|---|
| *Blood Factors* | |
| **Rh₀** ................ | D |
| **rh'** ................ | C |
| **rh''** ................ | E |
| **hr'** ................ | c |
| **hr''** ................ | e |
| **hr** ................ | f |
| *Rh Types* | |
| rh ................ | cde |
| rh' ................ | Cde |
| rh'' ................ | cdE |
| rhy ................ | CdE |
| Rh₀ ................ | cDe |
| Rh₁ ................ | CDe |
| Rh₂ ................ | cDE |
| Rhz ................ | CDE |

nomenclature by Allen and Rosenfield[25] consists of a numerical designation to indicate the observed serological reactions; thus a blood of type $Rh_1rh$ would be classified as $R^{1, 2-3, 4, 5}$. This nomenclature may suffice for genetic coding and statistical usage but precludes easy readability and clinical interpretation.

The Wiener Rh-Hr nomenclature,[22] presenting a logical sequence of symbols that are easily learned, leads to a better understanding of this complex blood group system. The Committee on Medicolegal Problems of the American Medical Association[26] has adopted the Rh-Hr nomenclature as the official terminology in medicolegal reports, and it has already been called the International Nomenclature in anticipation of its universal acceptance. As an aid to those who are not thoroughly familiar with this nomenclature the following conversion table may be consulted (see Table 4-III).

The possible errors that could result from the use of the C-D-E nomenclature is only one of the several reasons why the Rh-Hr nomenclature is preferable. The clear, logical and scientifically reasonable method for designating the Rh-Hr types is of fundamental importance to understanding this complex blood group system. This can be clearly demonstrated by comparing the Rh-Hr symbols for fifteen common phenotypes and the corresponding variations in the C-D-E system for the same types (Table 4-IV).

To summarize, the Wiener Rh-Hr nomenclature clearly indicates the indivisibility of the gene that determines the agglutinogen and in addition, emphasizes that the agglutinogen is recognized by its many blood factors, each of which is identified by its specific antibody. To avoid confusion in the spoken or written designation, the following convention is used:

1. The *gene*—an indivisible inherited unit on the chromosome, indicated by the use of italics and by the omission of the "h," while the symbol classification is printed as a superscript. Example: The agglutinogen rh′ is determined by the gene *r′* and the agglutinogen $Rh_1$ is determined by the gene *R′*.

2. The *agglutinogen*—the total Rh complex on the red cell,

TABLE 4-IV

THE Rh-Hr SYMBOLS FOR 15 COMMON PHENOTYPES AND SOME OF
THE CORRESPONDING SYMBOLS IN THE C-D-E NOMENCLATURE

| Rh-Hr | | C-D-E | | | | | |
|---|---|---|---|---|---|---|---|
| rh | = | cde/cde, | cde, | ccddee, | dccee, | | |
| rh'rh | = | Cde/cde, | Ccddee, | Ccdee, | dCcee, | | |
| rh'rh' | = | Cde/Cde, | CCddee, | CCdee, | dCCee, | | |
| rh"rh | = | cdE/cde, | ccdEe, | ccdEe, | dccEe, | | |
| rh"rh" | = | cdE/cdE, | ccddEE, | ccdEE, | dccEE, | | |
| rhy | = | Cde/cdE, | CcddEef, | CcdEef, | dCcEef, | | |
| rh'rh" | = | Cde/cdE, | CcddEe (f-), | CcdEe (f-), | dCcEe (f-), | | |
| Rh$_0$ | = | cDe, | cDee, | ccDee, | ccDDee, | Dcee, | Dccee |
| Rh$_1$rh | = | CDe/cde, | CDe/c-e, | CDe/cde, | CcDee, | CcDeef, | DCcee |
| Rh$_1$Rh$_1$ | = | CDe/CDe, | CDe/cDe, | cDe/Cde, | CCDdee, | CCDee, | DCCee |
| Rh$_1$Rh$_0$ | = | CDe/cDe, | CDe/C-e, | CCDDee, | CCDdee, | CcDeef, | DCcee |
| Rh$_2$Rh$_2$ | = | cDE/cDE, | cDe/cdE, | ccDDEE, | ccDEE, | cDE/c-e, | DccEE |
| Rh$_2$Rh$_0$ | = | cDE/cDe, | cDE/cdE, | ccDEe, | ccDEE, | cDE/c-E, | DccEe |
| Rh$_2$rh | = | cDE/cde, | CDe/cDE, | CcDdEe, | CcDEe, | DCcEe, | DccEe |
| Rh$_1$Rh$_2$ | = | CDe/cDE, | CDE/cde, | CcDdEef, | CcDEef, | DCcEef, | |
| | | CDe/cDE, | CDe/c-E, | CcDdEe (f-), | CcDEe (f-), | DCcEe (f-), | |

consisting of many blood factors. Printed in normal type—Rh₁rh.

3. The *antibody*—a serological substance which identifies and attaches to its specific agglutinogen. Example: anti-**Rh**$_0$. (Indicated by bold face)

4. The blood factor—one of the several serological specificities of the agglutinogen determined by its specific antibody. Example: **Rh**$_0$. (Indicated by bold face)

## Variants

The appearance of numerous alternative forms of the normal Rh antigens was explained by the multiple alleles that could exist at the Rh locus. As more reports of atypical findings were made, the nomenclature was expanded and became more complicated. However, with the Wiener Rh-Hr nomenclature, the new discoveries could be readily accommodated. The multiple allele theory permits any number of variations, whereas the Fisher-Race (C-D-E) system, because of inelasticity, was soon pressed into adding the concept of more loci and even overlooking some new findings.

Among the several new blood factors (the serological attributes of the Rh agglutinogen) that were discovered were some that are important because of their frequency, or their role in hemolytic disease of the newborn, or their part in transfusion reactions.

## ℜh$_0$ (**D**ᵘ)

This variant of Rh$_0$ was recognized when some anti-**Rh**$_0$ serums caused agglutination, while others did not.[27, 28] Cells carrying the ℜh$_0$ factor vary in their reactivity;[29] the variation being inherited. Some are agglutinated only by incomplete (univalent or blocking) serum; these are called "high grade" ℜh$_0$. Others require additional reinforcement with the antiglobulin test or with enzyme treatment; these are called "low grade" ℜh$_0$. It is of interest that a child who inherits the parent's variant, also inherits the "grade" of variant. Negroes possess the ℜh$_0$ variant more frequently than do Caucasians.

The determination of the presence of ℜh$_0$ is essential for clinical, genetic, and medicolegal reasons. A transfusion of blood containing this variant to a Rh-negative (rh) recipient can provoke the production of anti-$Rh_0$, exactly as if the recipient was infused with normal Rh-positive blood. Similarly, there have been reports of "low grade $\Re h_0$" persons who produced anti-$Rh_0$ when transfused with Rh-positive blood.[30] It has, therefore, been the practice among transfusionists to consider $\Re h_0$ ($D^u$) persons as Rh-negative when they are recipients and as Rh-positive when they are donors. Medicolegally, the need for definitely establishing the absence of the $\Re h_0$ factor in persons typed as Rh-negative (rh) is obvious, since this variant is an inherited characteristic.

A noninherited "weak" form of the $Rh_0$ blood factor was described by Ceppellini.[31, 32] He found the reaction with anti-$Rh_0$ serum was weaker if the gene determining $Rh_0$ was located on the chromosome opposite to one carrying the gene determining rh′. When the chromosome segregated separately in the next generation, this positional effect disappeared. This "weak" $Rh_0$ is not to be interpreted as true $\Re h_0$.

## Rh$^{ABCD}$

Other variations in the qualitative structure of the $Rh_0$ agglutinogen have been described by Wiener and collaborators.[33, 34] They investigated the rare finding of anti-$Rh_0$ antibodies in a person who was apparently $Rh_0$-positive. Such unusual serums agglutinated almost all $Rh_0$-positive cells except those of the donor. As explained, the $Rh_0$ agglutinogen consisted of several factors described as $Rh^A$, $Rh^B$, $Rh^C$, $Rh^D$, etc. If any of these factors are missing from the agglutinogen, it is possible that an exposure to Rh-positive red blood cells containing the missing factor would result in the production of an antibody against that specific component. Subsequently, any Rh-positive blood containing the complete $Rh_0$ agglutinogen would be agglutinated when tested with such serum. As more reports of these unusual "incomplete" agglutinogens[35, 36] appeared, it became obvious that the numerous combinations of blood factors involved in the Rh agglutinogen could only be explained by the Wiener multiple allele theory—since these atypical $Rh_0$ agglutinogens were also determined by inheritable genes.

### rh$^{w1}$ (formerly rh$^w$)

Further study of the Rh system soon revealed variants of the several other blood factors characterizing the Rh agglutinogen. Thus, rh′ could be separated into two subgroups when a new antibody, originally designated as anti-rh$^w$ (C$^w$) and now called anti-rh$^{w1}$ was described.[37] Although detected by most anti-rh′ serum, the blood factor rh$^{w1}$ could be selectively recognized by a pure anti-rh$^{w1}$ serum, which left the usual rh′ cells unagglutinated. Another less frequently encountered variation of the rh′ factor is rh$^{(')}$ (C$^u$)[38] which resembles $\mathfrak{Rh}_o$ (D$^u$) in requiring the antiglobulin test for identification. Still another rarer variant called rh′$^x$ (C$^x$) has been described only once.[39]

### rh$^{('')}$

The rh″ blood factor has also presented a variation described as rh$^{('')}$ (E$^u$).[40, 41] This variant is similar to Rh$_o$ and rh$^{(')}$ in being demonstrable only after the use of the specific serum (in this case anti-rh″) followed by the antiglobulin test. A rarer variant, named rh$^{w2}$ (E$^w$)[42] was found during the investigation of the causative antibody in a case of hemolytic disease of the newborn.

### hr$^s$

The antibody for this factor was described by Shapiro[43] and identifies a portion of the hr″ blood factor. Most anti-hr″ serums contain some anti-hr$^s$. However a pure anti-hr$^s$ serum might mistakenly be considered anti-hr″ unless tested against the rare hr″-positive cell lacking hr$^s$.

An error in determining the presence of hr″ might occur if pure anti-hr$^s$ serum is used, especially when testing the red blood cells of Negroes who occasionally lack hr$^s$ though having hr″. Wiener's nomenclature indicates hr″ positive cells lacking hr$^s$ by the use of a caret, for example, Rh$_2\hat{r}$h means reacting with anti-rh″ but not with anti-hr$^s$. This lack of hr$^s$, while rare, is an inherited characteristic and could be useful in medicolegal blood grouping.

## rh$^G$

A blood, negative with anti-**Rh**$_o$ and anti-**rh′** serums, was found to be positive with a compound serum called anti-**rh**$^G$.[44] It appears that almost all Rh$_o$-positive and rh′-positive persons also have the antigen **rh**$^G$. When an Rh-negative individual produces anti-**rh′**, then anti-**rh**$^G$ is also made along with the specific anti-**rh′**.

## hr

This unusual antibody, also known as "little f,"[45] identifies agglutinogens determined by the genes $R^o$ and $r$. Its greatest value lies in its ability to differentiate between the genotypes $R^1R^2$ and $R^zr$ and also between $r'r''$ and $r^yr$. This quality is especially useful in certain paternity blood grouping tests (Chapter Eight, Case #2449).

## rh$_i$

Among the several blood factors to which specific antiserums have been found is one called **rh**$_i$ (Ce),[46] which identifies the products of the gene complex $r'$ and $R^1$. Its usefulness lies in the ability to differentiate $r'r''$ from $r^yr$ as well as $R^1R^2$ from $R^zr$, the same quality as was demonstrated by anti-**hr** (f) serum.

## hr$^V$

Another serum of unusual specificity which reacts primarily with the blood of some Negroes carrying the genes $r$ or $R^o$ (**hr**-positive) is called anti-**hr**$^V$.[47] Approximately 25 percent of New York City Negroes are **hr**$^V$-positive. This serum provides a means of separating hr-positive red cells from Negroes into two subgroups, hr$^V$-negative and hr$^V$-positive.

Several other unusual variants in the Rh-Hr complex have been reported, many of scientific rather than clinical importance. Designation such as $r^M$,[48] $r^L$,[49] $e^i$,[50, 51] and $r'^N$ [52, 53] have been assigned to their gene determinants. In many instances their exact position in the Rh system is unclear.

### Deleted Genes or Super *Rh*$_o$

Under this unsatisfactory title are placed several unusual bloods which lack certain serological attributes of the normal Rh agglutinogens. Such bloods do not react with either anti-**rh′** or anti-**hr′** serum, nor with anti-**rh″** or anti-**hr″** serum. Its **Rh$_0$** component is exceptionally strong, enabling the agglutination of the cell in saline medium by univalent (conglutinating) anti-**Rh$_0$** serum. The original observers postulated a deletion of the chromosome bearing the Rh genes and designated its genotype as "—D—".[54, 55] An alternative explanation by Wiener[56] postulates an increased reactivity of the Rh$_0$ agglutinogen, crowding out the site of reactivity for the other blood factors. He indicated this gene complex as $\overset{=}{R}{}^o$ with a double bar, and the agglutinogen as $\overset{=}{\text{R}}\text{h}_0$ (Super Rh$_0$). Persons possessing this rare gene in the homozygous form are capable of producing a complex of antibodies against their several missing blood factors. Satisfactory crossmatching for transfusion is usually impossible unless persons of similar rare gene structure are available. Errors in paternity testing could easily occur unless the possibility of the presence of the rare $\overset{=}{R}{}^o$ gene is considered when exclusions based on the rh′-hr′ or rh″-hr″ relationship are found[57] (Chapter Eight, Case #2613).

An extremely rare phenotype, Rh null, lacking all Rh components[58] has been reported. It has been recognized only in the homozygous state, usually as a result of consanguinous matings. These unusual anomalies of the Rh agglutinogen such as $\overset{=}{\text{R}}\text{h}_0$ (lacking **rh′-hr′**, **rh″-hr″**), $\overset{-}{\text{R}}\text{h}_0$ (lacking only one of the **rh′-hr′**, **rh″-hr″** pairs), $\overset{-}{\text{R}}\text{h}^{\text{W}}$ (possessing **Rh$_0$** and **rh$^{\text{W1}}$** but lacking **rh′-hr′** and **rh″-hr″** etc.) are found only when an alert laboratory worker recognizes their atypical reactions. The thrill of discovery awaits those workers who pursue the investigation of such reactions, and the contribution they make to the subject of immunohematology is their just reward.

### Rh ANTISERUMS

The blood factors which characterize the Rh agglutinogen on the red cell act as antigens capable of provoking the production of antibodies when the red cell is injected into another human or animal lacking the antigen. The antibodies produced are specific for these antigens. Thus, an Rh-negative person injected with Rh$_0$-positive red cells will thereby be exposed to the **Rh$_0$** factor lacking from his own cells. He may, therefore, produce anti-**Rh$_0$**.

Should he then be reexposed to blood carrying the $Rh_0$ factor, the contact between his anti-**$Rh_0$** and the foreign $Rh_0$-positive blood will result in agglutination of the foreign red cells. *In vivo,* this produces a hemolytic transfusion reaction, since the foreign red cells are destroyed. If the sensitized person is female and pregnant with an $Rh_0$-positive fetus, the antibody can cross the placenta and destroy the unborn child's red blood cells if they have this antigen thus causing the disease erythroblastosis fetalis.[3]

As mentioned earlier, the original source of Rh testing serum was the immunized laboratory animal, either the rabbit or the guinea pig. Study of the antiserum produced in humans revealed it to be more reactive and far more abundant. At first the serum of accidentally immunized transfusion recipients was used. Soon the mothers of erythroblastotic infants became the source of large quantities of potent testing serums. A more controlled source was the deliberately immunized volunteer male donors who could be sensitized with carefully selected red cells to provide a "made-to-order" antiserum. Even this source proved barely adequate until the technic of plasmaphoresis was perfected. Using this method, 1,000 cc of plasma can be withdrawn weekly—the red cells being returned to the donor. Many of the rarer serums, however, must still be obtained from the patients where they were originally found, because the response to deliberate immunization with some of the rare blood factors is usually not satisfactory.

Since the antigenicity of the blood factors as well as the sensitivity of the donors differ, there is great variation in the quality, quantity, and the kind of antibody that is produced. Sometimes a single antibody will be made against a single blood factor of the agglutinogen, while at other times a polyvalent antiserum against a larger portion or against the entire agglutinogen will result. Thus, one may find anti-**$Rh_0$** only, or combinations such as anti-**$Rh_0$'** directed against both **$Rh_0$** and **rh'**. Occasionally, antibodies are found directed against agglutinogens having blood factors determined by the genes on only one of the pair of chromosomes (such as anti-**hr**, which react with **hr'** and **hr''** when they are results of the gene on a single chromosome). The multiple divisions of the Rh agglutinogens that can be differentiated by such complex serums are almost limitless. At present, at least twenty-eight phenotypes representing fifty-five geneotypes can be differentiated by such laboratory tests.

The kind of serum that can be produced also varies considerably. Some serums work best when tested against saline suspensions of the red cells. This was the usual testing medium before 1941. It soon became apparent that some antibodies could not be demonstrated by the classic saline method. Wiener showed the presence of such antibody activity by a "blocking" technic.[59] Shortly thereafter, a simpler method[60, 61, 62] using a colloidal medium, such as plasma or albumin, resulted in the visual agglutination of red cells by the blocking antibody. The original saline-acting antibody was at one time pictured as "bivalent," having two sites for the attachment to the red cells and therefore being large in size ($19S$ or $\gamma M$). The albumin-acting antibody was pictured as being "univalent," having only a single binding site and therefore being smaller in size ($7S$ or $\gamma G$). It is this latter "univalent" antibody that is capable of traversing the placenta and affecting susceptible fetal red cells. In 1945, a technic that was used years before in relation to bacterial tests was applied to the Rh antigen-antibody complex and found to be very effective. This test, called antihuman globulin or Coombs Test,[63, 64] was sensitive to extremely small amounts of different quality of antibody. It rapidly became a most valuable addition to the laboratory armamentarium and is presently the most frequently used means of performing compatibility tests for transfusion purposes.

Another discovery of importance was the finding that the pretreatment of the test cells with a proteolytic enzyme greatly increased the reactivity of the cells.[65, 66] Various enzymes including trypsin, ficin, papain, and bromelin are used for the purpose. Not all agglutinogens can be so enhanced however, since the proteolytic enzymes seem to damage the reacting sites for M-N-S, Kell and Duffy agglutinogens. An interesting combination of technics was described by Unger.[67] This consisted of the pretreatment of the red cells with a proteolytic enzyme to increase their reactivity, adding the specific testing serum to permit the antigen-antibody reaction to take place, and then reinforcing the reaction by the antiglobulin test. Using this method, several new agglutinogens were discovered.[68]

It is believed that other still undetected incompatibilities exist that are not exposed by any of these methods.[69] The search for the absolutely foolproof technic for blood grouping tests still awaits final success.

At present, each producer of antiserums supplies information on how best to use his particular product. These directions include the optimal conditions of temperature, duration of incubation, speed of centrifugation, and the need for fortification of the reaction with antiglobulin serum. These directions should be rigidly followed to obtain the optimal results.

For most laboratories concerned with blood typing, crossmatching, investigation of transfusion reactions and the study of erythroblastosis fetalis, the commercially available serums of specificities anti-**Rh**$_o$, anti-**rh'**, anti-**hr''**, anti-**hr'**, and anti-**hr''** are adequate. The use of a pool of human red blood cells having all the clinically important blood factors—also commercially available—permit the screening of recipients' and donors' blood for atypical antibodies. The presumptive identification of such antibodies requires the use of a panel of cells each containing a different combination of blood factors. Such panels are also available from the serum laboratories. The more complicated problems such as verification of the findings, the relationship to the rarer known antibodies or the identification of a "new" blood factor or antibody, require the facilities of a sophisticated research laboratory with its panels of rare antiserum and red cells with unusual blood factors. Such reference laboratories are located throughout the United States[70] and are always available for consultation.

## PITFALLS

The Rh-Hr blood groups which appeared to be relatively simple in 1941 have evolved into a most complex system. The intensive study following its discovery has uncovered a series of variants, suppressions, deletions, and weak reactions—all demanding caution and understanding when performing Rh groupings, crossmatchings or testing for medicolegal purposes. Pitfalls for the unwary exist in many areas; these require special attention.

$\mathfrak{Rh}_o$

The presence of these variants can be determined by the use of an incomplete antiserum (having $\gamma$ G **Rh**$_o$ antibodies) followed by the antihuman globulin test. The anti-**Rh**$_o$ serum must have been tested and proven capable of recognizing such variants. Failure to agglutinate in the first step (serum plus cells) with agglutination visible in the second step (after addition of the antihuman globulin) identifies the $\mathfrak{Rh}_o$ factors. Another technic requires the use of a very high titer, high protein anti-**Rh**$_o$ univalent or incomplete serum enhanced by high speed centrifugation.[71]

As mentioned earlier, persons with the variant $\mathfrak{Rh}_o$ agglutinogen are treated as Rh-negative when they are recipients of blood transfusions and as Rh-positive when they are donors. The determination of the presence of the variant is also useful medicolegally since it is an inherited characteristic.

### Rh$_o$ With Anti-Rh$_o$

This apparent paradox is explained by the absence of some of the normal **Rh**$_o$ blood factors that make up the standard Rh$_o$ agglutinogen. The production of antibodies against the missing factor results in an antiserum which will agglutinate all Rh-positive bloods except those bloods missing the same factors. Several of the specificities of the Rh$_o$ agglutinogen have been identified and named **Rh**$^A$, **Rh**$^B$, **Rh**$^C$, and so forth.[33, 34]

### Super Rh$_o$—$\overline{\overline{\text{Rh}}}_o$

The Rh agglutinogen which lacks all trace of the normally expected **rh'**, **hr'**, **rh''**, **hr''** factors is of importance in crossmatching of blood for transfusion purposes and in parentage studies. The serum usually contains a complex of antibodies against many of the missing blood factors—this makes donor procurement for transfusion almost impossible. Such problems can only be solved by obtaining a donor of similar phenotype; most usually found among the patient's siblings. Several such units of blood have been stored in the frozen state* and are available for emergencies.

---

* U.S.N.H. Chelsea, Massachusetts and the Greater N. Y. Blood Center, N. Y. C.

This variant is suspected when the tests with antiserum **rh′**, **hr′**, **rh″**, and **hr″** are negative, contrary to the rule of reciprocal relationships. The final proof of this finding is the agglutination of a *saline* suspension of the suspect cell by incomplete (univalent) anti-**Rh**$_0$ serum and by titration and scoring.[72] The danger of erroneous exclusion of parentage exists unless this possibility is considered and the necessary tests included before conclusions based on rh′-hr′ and rh″-hr″ relationship are finalized. Several such cases have already been reported.[5, 73, 74]

An extremely rare instance, where the strong $\overline{\text{Rh}}_0$ agglutinogen lacked only the blood factors **rh″** and **hr″**, has been found.[75] The symbol $\overline{\text{Rh}}_0$ (with a single bar) has been assigned to this variant. No example of blood lacking only the pair **rh′-hr′** has yet been found.

### rh$^{(′)}$, rh$^{(″)}$

These extremely rare variants, which resemble $\mathfrak{R}\text{h}_0$ by requiring the use of the antihuman globulin test to fortify the reaction between the antigen and the corresponding antibody, are inheritable characteristics. In parentage exclusions where an apparently homozygous parent (**hr″**-negative) fails to transmit an **rh″** factor to the child, the antihuman globulin test should be performed on the negative reaction. The same situation could exist with the **rh′-hr′** relationship. "Pure" anti-**rh′** or anti-**rh″** serum must be used if the antihuman globulin test is to follow, since the usual "blocked" serum will give false positive reactions due to the anti-**Rh**$_0$ which is present.

### hr′, hr″

The test for the Hr factors provide indirect evidence about the zygosity of the **rh′** and **rh″** blood factors. If the tests are negative, they infer that **rh′** and **rh″** are present in the homozygous state. Such inferences, especially in Negroes, should be carefully considered. Additional steps must be taken to verify these conclusions. Among the useful technics to achieve valid results are the following:

1. $\overline{\overline{\text{Rh}}}_0$—A *saline* suspension of the red cells is tested with an incomplete (univalent) anti-**Rh**$_0$ serum adjusted to give

a negative reaction with saline suspended normal cells.

2. **rh′** and **rh″**—The negative reaction between the test cell and "pure" (not blocked) anti-**rh′** or anti-**rh″** serum is converted to the antihuman globulin test.

3. **hr′** and **hr″**—The presence of a single or double dose of a blood factor (homozygous or heterozygous state) can frequently be determined by the use of a titration and scoring technic.[72] A suspected reaction can be verified by elution of the attached antibody and testing the eluate against the appropriate cells.[76, 77, 78]

4. **hr**—The antiserum for blood factor **hr** is useful to differentiate between the phenotypes $Rh_1Rh_2$ and $Rh_zrh$, and between rh′rh″ and $rh_yrh$. This test can be very valuable in paternity matters especially in Caucasians where the frequency of these blood types ($Rh_1Rh_2$) is approximately 13 percent.

## MEDICOLEGAL ASPECTS

The Rh-Hr blood group system has greatly increased the usefulness of blood grouping tests for medicolegal purposes. In disputed paternity tests, 25 percent of falsely accused men can be excluded by this system alone. The tests, however, are highly sophisticated and the proper use of the information obtained from the tests requires a sound understanding of the basic genetics, familiarity with the variants, and a knowledge of the technics necessary for their demonstration. It is important that all parties involved be tested with the same lot of serum and also simultaneously, if practicable. Interpretation of the results of the blood test of Negroes require careful consideration before final conclusions are made; especially regarding the reactions with anti-**hr′** and anti-**hr″** serums.

Having established the correct Rh-Hr groupings of each of the parties in the case, the use of Table 4-V may facilitate the final conclusion. This table enables a rapid method of indicating those children that could not result from each set of matings. The table indicates (by normal type) those Rh-Hr groups of children for whom paternity is excluded; it also indicates (by boldface type) those for whom maternity is excluded. This con-

## TABLE 4-V

### Exclusion of Paternity by the Rh-Hr Blood Types*

| | | Phenotype of Putative Father | | | | |
|---|---|---|---|---|---|---|
| | | 1 | 2 | 3 | 4 | 5 |
| Phenotype of Putative Mother | | rh $Rh_o$ | rh'rh $Rh_1$rh | rh'rh' $Rh_1Rh_1$ | rh''rh $Rh_2$rh | rh''rh'' $Rh_2Rh_2$ |
| 1 | rh $Rh_o$ | 2, **3**, 4, **5**, **6a**, 6b, 7, 8, 9 | **3**, 4, **5**, **6a**, 6b, 7, 8, 9 | 1, **3**, 4, **5**, 6a, 6b, 7, 8, 9 | 2, **3**, **5**, **6a**, 6b, 7, 8, 9 | 1, 2, **3**, **5**, **6a**, 6b, 7, 8, 9 |
| 2 | rh'rh $Rh_1Rh$ | 3, 4, **5**, 6a, 6b, 7, **8**, 9 | 4, **5**, 6a, 6b, 6b, 7, **8**, 9 | 1, 4, **5**, 6a, 6b, 7, **8**, 9 | 3, **5**, 6b, 7, **8**, 9 | 1, 2, 3, **5**, 6b, 7, **8**, 9 |
| 3 | rh'rh' $Rh_1Rh_1$ | **1**, 3, **4**, **5**, 6a, **6b**, 7, **8**, 9 | **1**, **4**, **5**, 6a, **6b**, 7, **8**, 9 | **1**, 2, **4**, **5**, 6a, **6b**, 7, **8**, 9 | **1**, 3, **4**, **5**, **6b**, 7, **8**, 9 | **1**, 2, 3, **4**, **5**, **6b**, 7, **8**, 9 |
| 4 | rh''rh $Rh_2Rh$ | 2, **3**, 5, 6a, 6b, **7**, 8, 9 | **3**, 5, 6b, **7**, 8, 9 | 1, **3**, 4, 5, 6b, **7**, 8, 9 | 2, **3**, 6a, 6b, **7**, 8, 9 | 1, 2, **3**, 6a, 6b, **7**, 8, 9 |
| 5 | rh''rh'' $Rh_2Rh_2$ | **1**, **2**, **3**, 5, 6a, **6b**, 7, 8, 9 | **1**, **2**, **3**, 5, 6b, 7, 8, 9 | **1**, **2**, **3**, 4, 5, **6b**, 7, 8, 9 | **1**, **2**, **3**, 6a, **6b**, 7, 8, 9 | **1**, **2**, **3**, 4, 6a, **6b**, 7, 8, 9 |
| 6a | rh'rh'' $Rh_1Rh_2$ | **1**, 3, 5, 6a, **6b**, 7, 8, 9 | **1**, 5, **6b**, 7, 8, 9 | **1**, 2, 4, 5, **6b**, 7, 8, 9 | **1**, 3, **6b**, 7, 8, 9 | **1**, 2, 3, 4, **6b**, 7, 8, 9 |
| 6b | rhyrh $Rh_zRh_o$ | 2, **3**, 4, **5**, **6a**, 7, 8, 9 | **3**, 4, **5**, **6a**, 8, 9 | 1, **3**, 4, **5**, **6a**, 6b, 8, 9 | 2, **3**, **5**, **6a**, 7, 9 | 1, 2, **3**, **5**, **6a**, 6b, 7, 9 |
| 7 | rhyrh' $Rh_zRh_1$ | **1**, 3, **4**, **5**, 6a, 7, 8, 9 | **1**, **4**, **5**, 6a, 8, 9 | **1**, 2, **4**, **5**, 6a, 6b, 8, 9 | **1**, 3, **4**, **5**, 7, 9 | **1**, 2, 3, **4**, **5**, 6b, 7. 9 |
| 8 | rhyrh'' $Rh_zRh_2$ | **1**, **2**, **3**, 5, 6a, 7, 8, 9 | **1**, **2**, **3**, 5, 8, 9 | **1**, **2**, **3**, 4, 5, 6b, 8, 9 | **1**, **2**, **3**, 6a, 7, 9 | **1**, **2**, **3**, 4, 6a, 6b, 7, 9 |
| 9 | rhyrhy $Rh_zRh_z$ | **1**, **2**, **3**, **4**, **5**, **6a**, 7, 8, 9 | **1**, **2**, **3**, **4**, **5**, **6a**, 8, 9 | **1**, **2**, **3**, **4**, **5**, **6a**, 6b, 8, 9 | **1**, **2**, **3**, **4**, **5**, **6b**, 7, 9 | **1**, **2**, **3**, **4**, **5**, **6a**, 6b, 7, 9 |

Underlined bold face figures represent phenotypes of children for whom maternity is excluded.

This table is to be applied only to matings in which at least one of the parents is $Rh_o$ positive. Where both parents are $RH_o$ negative, necessarily all $RH_o$ positive children are excluded.

The phenotypes corresponding to the code numbers are given in the marginal headings, e.g. 1 is the code number for phenotypes rh and $Rh_o$

*From A. S. Wiener with permission of author.

= Bold Face = phenotypes of children from whom **maternity** is excluded.

Where both parents are $RH_o$ negative, all $RH_o$ positive children are necessarily excluded.

This table is to be applied only where at least one parent is $Rh_o$ positive.

Each code no. corresponds to a phenotype in the marginal headings, e.g. 1 is the code no. for phenotype rh and Rh

TABLE 4-V (continued)

| Phenotype of Putative Father | | | | |
|---|---|---|---|---|
| 6a | 6b | 7 | 8 | 9 |
| rh'rh" | rhyrh | rhyrh' | rhyrh" | rhyrhy |
| Rh₁Rh₂ | RhzRho | RhzRh₁ | RhzRh₂ | RhzRhz |
| 1, **3, 5, 6a,** 6b, 7, 8, 9 | 2, 3, 4, 5, 6a, 7, 8, 9 | 1, 3, 4, 5, 6a, 7, 8, 9 | 1, 2, 3, 5, 6a, 7, 8, 9 | 1, 2, 3, 4, 5, 6a, 7, 8, 9 |
| 1, 5 6b, 7, 8, 9 | 3, 4, 5, 6a, 8, 9 | 1, 4, 5, 6a, 8, 9 | 1, 2, 3, 5, 8, 9 | 1, 2, 3, 4, 5, 6a, 8, 9 |
| 1, 2, 4, 5, 6b, 7, 8, 9 | 1, 3, 4, 5, 6a, 6b, 8, 9 | 1, 2, 4, 5, 6a, 6b, 8, 9 | 1, 2, 3, 4, 5, 6b, 8, 9 | 1, 2, 3, 4, 5, 6a, 6b, 8, 9 |
| 1, 3, 6b, 7, 8, 9 | 2, 3, 5, 6a, 7, 9 | 1, 3, 4, 5, 7, 9 | 1, 2, 3, 6a 7, 9 | 1, 2, 3, 4, 5, 6a, 7, 9 |
| 1, 2, 3, 4, 6b, 7, 8, 9 | 1, 2, 3, 5, 6a, 6b, 7, 9 | 1, 2, 3, 4, 5, 6b, 7, 9 | 1, 2, 3, 4, 6a, 6b, 7, 9 | 1, 2, 3, 4, 5, 6a, 6b, 7, 9 |
| 1, 2, 4, 6b, 7, 8, 9 | 1, 3, 5, 6a, 6b, 9 | 1, 2, 4, 5, 6b, 9 | 1, 2, 3, 4, 6b, 9 | 1, 2, 3, 4, 5, 6a, 6b, 9 |
| 1, 3, 5, 6a, 6b, 9 | 2, 3, 4, 5, 6a, 7, 8 | 1, 3, 4, 5, 6a, 8 | 1, 2, 3, 5, 6a, 7 | 1, 2, 3, 4, 5, 6a, 7, 8 |
| 1, 2, 4, 5, 6b, 9 | 1, 3, 4, 5, 6a, 8 | 1, 2, 4, 5, 6a, 6b, 8 | 1, 2, 3, 4, 5, 6b, | 1, 2, 3, 4, 5, 6a, 6b, 8 |
| 1, 2, 3, 4, 6b, 9 | 1, 2, 3, 5, 6a, 7 | 1, 2, 3, 4, 5, 6b | 1, 2, 3, 4, 6a, 6b, 7 | 1, 2, 3, 4, 5, 6a, 6b, 7 |
| 1, 2, 3, 4, 5, 6a, 6b, 9 | 1, 2, 3, 4, 5, 6a, 7, 8 | 1, 2, 3, 4, 5, 6a, 6b, 8 | 1, 2, 3, 4, 5, 6a, 6b, 7 | 1, 2, 3, 4, 5, 6a, 6b, 7, 8 |

cise table replaces many pages of notations which give the same information.

Basically the fundamental laws of inheritance in the Rh-Hr system are simple and similar to the laws governing the A-B-O and M-N-S systems.

1. A blood factor cannot appear in the blood of a child unless present in one or both parents.

2. A parent who is homozygous for a blood factor must transmit a gene for this factor to his child.

3. A child who is homozygous for a blood factor must have inherited a gene for this factor from each of its parents.

The usefulness of this system is not limited to exclusion of parentage. Its application to problems of identification, "mixed babies," kidnapped children,[79] and derivative citizenship[80] have enabled the just and proper settlement of many such issues. Several examples of the use of the Rh-Hr system in such situations are presented in Chapter Eight.

The Rh-Hr blood group system, whose discovery stimulated the new science of immunohematology, has proved to be of great clinical and forensic importance. Blood transfusions have been made safer, the rational treatment of erythroblastotic infants has greatly reduced the mortality from the disease, and the application of the principles of heredity has permitted the resolution of many problems in paternity disputes, mixed baby cases, derivative citizenship, and similar problems. Understanding the genetics and technics of this system provides the immunohematologists with a most valuable tool, not only in the management of clinical conditions, but also in application to medicolegal problems.

## REFERENCES

1. Landsteiner, K., and Wiener, A. S.: An agglutinable factor in human blood recognized by immune sera from rhesus blood. *Proc. Soc. Exper. Biol. & Med.*, 43:223, 1940.

2. Wiener, A. S., and Peters, H. R.: Hemolytic reactions following transfusion of blood of homologous group, with three cases in which the same agglutinogen was responsible. *Ann. Int. Med.*, 13:2306, 1940.

3. Levine, P., Burnham, L., Katzin, E. M., and Vogel, P.: The role of iso-immunization in the pathogenesis of erythroblastosis fetalis. *Am. J. Obst. & Gynec.*, 42:925, 1941.

4. Landsteiner, K., and Wiener, A. S.: Studies on an agglutinogen (Rh) in human blood reacting with anti-rhesus sera and with human isoantibodies. *J. Exper. Med.*, 74:309, 1941.

5. Race, R. R., and Sanger, R.: *Blood Groups in Man.* 5th ed. Philadelphia, F. A. Davis Co., 1968, p. 171.

6. Wiener, A. S.: *Rh-Hr Blood Types.* New York, Grune & Stratton, 1954.

7. Wiener, A. S.: *An Rh-Hr Syllabus.* New York, Grune & Stratton, 1954.

8. Weiner, A. S., and Wexler, I. B.: *Heredity of the Blood Groups.* New York, Grune & Stratton, 1958.

9. Boorman, K. E., and Dodd, B. E.: *Blood Group Serology.* 3d ed. Boston, Little, Brown & Co., 1966.

10. Erskine, A. G.: *The Principles and Practice of Blood Grouping.* St. Louis, Mosby & Co., 1973.

11. Wiener, A. S.: Hemolytic reaction following transfusions of blood of homologous group; further observations on role of property Rh particularly in cases without demonstrable isoantibodies. *Arch. Path., 32:*227, 1941.

12. Wiener, A. S., and Landsteiner, K.: Heredity of variants of Rh type. *Proc. Soc. Exper. Biol. & Med., 53:*167, 1943.

13. Wiener, A. S.: Distribution and heredity of variants of Rh types. *Science, 98:*182, 1943.

14. Wiener, A. S., and Sonn, E. B.: Additional variants of Rh type demonstrable with special human anti-Rh serum. *J. Immunol., 47:*461, 1943.

15. Wiener, A. S.: Genetic theory of the Rh blood types. *Proc. Soc. Exper. Biol. & Med., 54:*316, 1943.

16. Levine, P.: The pathogenesis of erythroblastosis fetalis. *J. Ped., 23:*656, 1943.

17. Race, R. R., and Taylor, G. L.: Serum that discloses genotype of Rh-positive people. *Nature,* London, *152:*300, 1943.

18. Mourant, A. E.: A new rhesus antibody. *Nature,* London, *155:*542, 1945.

19. Wiener, A. S., and Peters, H. R.: Intragroup incompatibility due to hr″ factor. *Am. J. Clin. Path., 18:*533, 1948.

20. Mourant, A. E.: *Distribution of the Human Blood Groups.* Oxford, Blackwell Scientific Publishers, 1954.

21. Wiener, A. S.: Genetic theory of the Rh blood types. *Proc. Soc. Exper. Biol. & Med., 54:*316, 1943.

22. Wiener, A. S.: Nomenclature of Rh blood types. *Science, 99:*532, 1944.

23. Race, R. R.: The Rh genotypes and Fisher's theory. *Blood,* v.3, spec. issue #2: p. 27, 1948.

24. Lawler, S. D., Bertinshaw, D., Sanger, R., and Race, R. R.: Inheritance of Rh blood groups: 150 families tested with anti-C, -c, -C$^w$, -D, -E and anti-e. *Ann. Eugenics, 15:*258, 1950.

25. Rosenfield, R. E., Allen, F. H., Jr., Swisher, S. N., and Kochwa, S.: A review of Rh serology and presentation of a new terminology. *Transfusion, 2:*287, 1962.

26. Owen, R. D., Stormont, C., Wexler, I. B., and Wiener, A. S.: Medicolegal applications of blood-grouping tests. *J.A.M.A., 164:*2036, 1957.

27. Stratton, F.: A new Rh allelomorph. *Nature,* London, *158:*25, 1946.

28. Race, R. R., Sanger, R., and Lawler, S. D.: Rh genes allelomorphic to D. *Nature*, London, *163*:292, 1948.

29. Bush, M., Sabo, B., Siroup, M., and Masouredis, S. P.: Red cell D antigen sites and titration scores in a family with weak and normal $D^u$ phenotypes inherited from a homozygous $D^u$ mother. *Transfusion, 14*:433, 1974.

30. Argall, C. I., Ball, J. M., and Trentelman, E.: Presence of anti-D antibody in the serum of a $D^u$ patient. *J. Lab & Clin. Med., 41*:895, 1953.

31. Ceppellini, R., Dunn, L. C., and Turri, M.: An interaction between alleles at the Rh locus in man which weakens the reactivity of the $Rh_0$ factor ($D^u$). *Proc. Nat. Acad. Sci., 41*:283, 1955.

32. Masouredes, S. P., and Sturgeon, P.: Quantitative serologic and isotopic studies on the $Rh_0$ variant—$D^u$. *Blood, 25*:954, 1965.

33. Wiener, A. S., Geiger, J., and Gordon, E. B.: Mosaic nature of the $Rh_0$ factor of human blood. *Exper. Med. & Surg., 15*:75, 1957.

34. Unger, L. J., and Wiener, A. S.: Some observations on blood factors $Rh^A$, $Rh^B$, and $Rh^C$ of the Rh-Hr blood group system. *Blood, 14*:522, 1959.

35. Sacks, M. S., Wiener, A. S., Jahn, E. F., Spurling, C. L., and Unger, L. J.: Isosensitization to the new blood factor $Rh^D$ with special reference to its clinical importance. *Ann. Int. Med., 51*:740, 1959.

36. Sussman, L. N., and Wiener, A. S.: An unusual Rh agglutinogen lacking blood factors **$Rh^A$**, **$Rh^B$**, **$Rh^C$**, and **$Rh^D$**. *Transfusion, 4*:50, 1964.

37. Callender, S. T., and Race, R. R.: A serological and genetical study of multiple antibodies formed in response to blood transfusion by a patient with lupus erythematosis diffusus. *Ann. Eugenics, 13*:102, 1946.

38. Race, R., Sanger, R., and Lawler, S. D.: Rh genes allelomorphic to C. *Nature*, London, *161*:316, 1948.

39. Stratton, F., and Renton, P. H.: Haemolytic disease of the newborn caused by a new Rh antibody, anti-$C^x$. *Brit. Med. J. 1*:962, 1954.

40. Ceppellini, R., Ikin, E. W., and Mourant, A. E.: A new allele of the Rh gene E. *Boll. Ist. Siero, Milanese, 29*:123, 1950.

41. Sussman, L. N.: The rare blood factor **$rh^{(\prime\prime)}$** or $E^u$. *Blood, 10*:1241, 1955.

42. Greenwalt, T. J., and Sanger, R.: The Rh antigen $E^w$. *Brit. J. Haemat., 1*:52, 1955.

43. Shapiro, M.: Serology and genetics of a new blood factor: $hr^S$. *J. Forensic Med., 7*:96, 1960.

44. Allen, F. H. Jr., and Tippett, P. A.: A new Rh blood type which reveals the Rh antigen G. *Vox Sanguinis, 3*:321, 1958.

45. Sanger, R., Race, R. R., Rosenfield, R. E., Vogel, P., and Gibbel, N.:

Anti-f and the "new" Rh antigen it defines. *Proc. Nat. Acad. Sci.,* 39:824, 1953.

46. Rosenfield, R. E., and Haber, G. V.: An Rh blood factor, $rh_i$(Ce), and its relationship to hr(ce). *Am. J. Human Genet.* 10:474, 1958.

47. DeNatale, A., Cahan, A., Jack, J. A., Race, R. R., and Sanger, R.: V, a "new" Rh antigen, common in negroes, rare in white people. *J.A.M.A., 159:*247, 1955.

48. Tippett, P. A., Sanger, R., Dunsford, I., and Barber, M.: An Rh gene complex $r^M$, in some ways like $r^G$. *Vox Sanguinis,* 6:21, 1961.

49. Metaxas, M. N., and Metaxas-Buhler, M.: An Rh gene complex which produces weak c and e antigens in a mother and her son. *Vox Sanguinis,* 6:136, 1961.

50. Layrisse, M., Layrisse, Z., Garcia, E., Wilbert, J., and Parra, R. J.: A new Rh phenotype $Dcce^ie^if$ found in a chibcha Indian tribe. *Nature,* London, *191:*503, 1961.

51. Layrisse, M., Layrisse, Z., Garcia, E., and Parra, J.: Genetic studies of the new Rh chromosome $Dce^if$ ($Rh_o{}^i$) found in a chibcha tribe. *Vox Sanguinis,* 6:710, 1961.

52. Sturgeon, P., Fisk, R., Wintler, C., and Chertok, R.: *Observations with Pure Anti-C on a Variant of C Common in Negroes.* Proc. 7th Congress of the International Society of Blood Transfusion, held in Rome in 1958. Published by S. Karger (Basel) in 1958, p. 293.

53. Sturgeon, P.: Studies on the relation of anti-rh′$^N$ ($C^N$) to Rh blood factor $rh_i$ (Ce). *J. Forensic Sci.,* 5:287, 1960.

54. Race, R. R., Sanger, R., and Selwyn, J. G.: Probable deletion in human Rh chromosome. *Nature,* London, *166:*520, 1950.

55. Race, R. R., Sanger, R., and Selwyn, J. G.: Possible deletion in human Rh chromosome: a serological and genetical study. *Brit. J. Exper. Path.,* 32:124, 1951.

56. Wiener, A. S., Gordon, E. B., and Cohen, L.: A new rare rhesus agglutinogen. *Am. J. Human Genet.,* 4:363, 1952.

57. Wiener, A. S., Unger, L. J., and Sacks, M. S.: Rh-Hr blood types—present status. Report of the Committee on Medicolegal Problems of the American Medical Association. *J.A.M.A., 172:*1158, 1960.

58. Vos, G. H., Vos, D., Kirk, R. L., and Sanger, R.: A sample of blood with no detectable Rh antigens. *Lancet, 1:*14, 1961.

59. Wiener, A. S.: A new test (blocking test) for Rh sensitization. *Proc. Soc. Exper. Biol. & Med.,* 56:173, 1944.

60. Race, R. R.: An "incomplete" antibody in human serum. *Nature,* London, *153:*771, 1944.

61. Diamond, L. K., and Abelson, N. M.: The importance of Rh inhibitor substance in anti-Rh serums. *J. Clin. Invest.,* 24:122, 1945.

62. Wiener, A. S.: Conglutination test for Rh sensitization. *J. Lab. & Clin. Med., 30:*662, 1945.

63. Coombs, R. R. A., Mourant, A. E., and Race, R. R.: Detection of weak and "incomplete" Rh agglutinins: A new test. *Lancet, 2:*15, 1945.

64. Dunsford, I., and Grant, J.: *The Antiglobulin (Coombs) Test in Laboratory Practice.* London, Oliver and Boyd, 1960.

65. Pickles, M. M.: Effect of cholera filtrate on red cells as demonstrated by incomplete Rh antibodies. *Nature,* London, *158:*880, 1946.

66. Wiener, A. S., and Katz, L.: Studies on the use of enzyme treated red cells in tests for Rh sensitization. *J. Immunol., 66:*51, 1951.

67. Unger, L. J.: A method for detecting $Rh_0$ antibodies in extremely low titer. *J. Lab. & Clin. Med., 37:*825, 1951.

68. Unger, L. J., and Katz, L.: The effect of trypsin on hemagglutinogens determining eight blood group systems. *J. Lab. & Clin. Med. 39:* 135, 1952.

69. Walker, P. C., Jennings, E. R., and Monroe, C.: Hemolytic transfusion reaction after the administration of apparently compatible blood. *Amer. J. Clin. Path., 44:*193, 1965.

70. American Association of Blood Banks, Central Office, Suite 1322, 30 N. Michigan Ave., Chicago, Ill. 60602. Membership Roster.

71. Sturgeon, P.: The $Rh_0$ variant—$D^u$: II—Its detection with a direct tube test. *Transfusion, 2:*244, 1962.

72. Sussman, L. N.: Titration and scoring in disputed parentage. *Transfusion, 5:*248, 1965.

73. Henningsen, K.: Significance of D-chromosome in a legal paternity case. *Vox Sanguinis, 2:*399, 1957.

74. Broman, B., and Heiken, A.: Further instances of possible mutations affecting the Rh blood group system. *Hereditas, 48:*307, 1962.

75. Tate, H., Cunningham, C., McDade, M. G., Tippett, P. A., and Sanger, R.: An Rh gene complex Dc-. *Vox Sanguinis, 5:*398, 1960.

76. Jensen, K. G.: Elution of incomplete antibodies from red cells. A comparison of different methods. *Vox Sanguinis, 4:*230, 1959.

77. Rubin, H.: Antibody elution from red blood cells. *J. Clin. Path., 16:*70, 1963.

78. Sussman, L. N., and Pretshold, H.: Elution technic for identification of antibody-coated erythrocytes. *Am. J. Clin. Path., 24:*1430, 1954.

79. Wiener, A. S.: Application of blood grouping tests in cases of disputed maternity. *J. Forensic Sci., 4:*351, 1959.

80. Sussman, L. N.: Application of blood grouping to derivative citizenship. *J. Forensic Sci., 1:*101, 1956.

CHAPTER FIVE

# THE KELL AND OTHER BLOOD GROUP SYSTEMS

Leon N. Sussman

## THE KELL SYSTEM

THE ROUTINE USE of the antihuman globulin test, introduced in 1945, led to the discovery of several new blood group systems. The first of these was described in 1946[1] when a previously unidentified antibody was found in the serum of the mother of a child with erythroblastosis fetalis. This antibody was not related to the A-B-O, M-N, or Rh systems. It did agglutinate the red blood cells of the father and a sibling of the affected infant. The antigen was called Kell after the name of the family in whom it was found, and it was assigned the designation "K." A second example was found independently shortly thereafter.[2] This one had caused a severe hemolytic transfusion reaction.

Family studies revealed that the **Kell** factor was inherited as a dominant Mendelian character. It was present in about 7 percent of Caucasians, rare in Negroids, and absent in Mongoloids. Many examples of this antibody have since been found—demonstrated best by the use of the antihuman globulin test and/or the conglutination test.

The discovery of the allele of *K*, named *k*, by Levine[3] in 1949, seemingly completed the K-k system. This permitted population studies that corroborated the theory of inheritance. Thereafter, the system was outlined as follows:

homozygous *KK* with a frequency of 0.12 percent
heterozygous *Kk* with a frequency of 6.75 percent
the frequent recessive *kk* with a frequency of 93.12 percent

The antigenicity of the **Kell** factor approximates that of the **hr′** factor; however, because of its lower frequency, there is less

87

opportunity for sensitization to take place. Nevertheless, the possibility that a transfusion reaction or hemolytic disease of the newborn could result from sensitization to the **Kell** factor must always be considered. For this reason a person who is known to have anti-**Kell** must be transfused with K-negative blood only; and an erythroblastotic infant of a mother who has anti-**Kell** must be treated with K-negative blood only.

It was not until 1957 that other antigens related to the Kell system were reported. These new factors were designated **Kp**[a 4] and **Kp**[b].[5] Their antiserums are very rare. Further investigations of the Kell group yielded some evidence of very rare people (frequency .006%) with no Kell antigens, called K$_o$.[6] Further addition to the Kell group was the finding that the antigen Js[a] and Js[b] belonged to the system and were particularly useful in discriminating between Negroes[7] where Js[a] positive people have a frequency of 15 to 20 percent. The genetics of the K-k system now is assuming the complexities of the A-B-O and Rh-Hr blood groups.

In paternity testing, the most useful antigens in this system are K for Caucasians and Js[a] for Negroes because of their unusual frequency.

For medicolegal purposes, the Kell system has usefulness in the hands of qualified experts who have the serums available. Many commercial serum laboratories do have anti-**Kell** and occasionally anti-**Js**[a]. At present, the chief practical application of this system lies in the unequivocal exclusion of paternity that exists when a child is found to be Kell-positive, and both the mother and the alleged father are Kell-negative. A similar exclusion exists as first order exclusion in the Js[a] system; that is, a positive Js[a] child cannot have a negative mother and a negative alleged father. The law of inheritance states that a blood factor cannot be present in the blood of a child unless it is present in the blood of either the mother or the father.

Examples of Exclusion of Paternity:

| Putative Father | A | MN | Rh$_o$ | K-negative |
|---|---|---|---|---|
| Mother | B | M | Rh$_o$ | K-negative |
| Infant | O | M | Rh$_o$ | K-positive |

An exclusion of paternity is present in that the child is Kell-positive, whereas the mother and the alleged father are both Kell-negative.

The Kell system, utilizing anti-**K** for Caucasians and anti-**Js**[a] for Negroes, while not approved for routine use in medicolegal situations, should be incorporated into blood grouping tests. Qualified experts, using proper controls and with a full understanding of the genetics involved, may submit their findings to the court when an exclusion is found.

## OTHER BLOOD GROUP SYSTEMS

Several other blood group systems are recognized as being independent of the A-B-O, M-N, Rh-Hr, and Kell blood groups. When a blood group system is characterized by an agglutinogen which is found in more than 5 percent of the population, it is considered a "public" system. These additional public systems are of scientific importance but clinically they are not usually significant, since neither their frequency nor their antigenicity approaches that of the blood group systems already described. Antiserums to detect their blood factors are not common, being ordinarily found only in large blood centers or research laboratories. A short résumé of these groups follows; for those interested in more details, reference should be made to the original articles describing the system and to the several standard texts already quoted.

### The P System

The production of anti-**M** and anti-**N** serum in the immunized rabbits was accompanied by the finding of another antibody in the rabbit serum to which was assigned the name anti-**P**.[8] The same antibody was subsequently made in other animals. It is also found both as a natural and immune antibody in man. It is classified as a "cold" antibody, being most active at or below 20°C. The **P** factor is found most frequently in Negroids (98%), less frequently in Caucasians (78%), and least frequently in Mongoloids (30%). The antigen is inherited as a simple Mendelian dominant.[9] Differences in reactivity of the various examples of anti-**P**, and its weak or absent reaction at body temperature has made the P system of little clinical or medicolegal significance. Interest in this system again became acute when it was shown[10] that a rare antibody (anti-$Tj^a$) described by Levine[11] in 1951, belonged to the P system. Three allelic genes were postulated $P^1$, $P^2$, and $p$. The rare $p$ gene determined the Tj(a−) blood that was capable of producing both anti-**P** and anti-$Tj^a$; the $P^2$ gene determining the P-negative blood, capable of producing only anti-$P^1$; and the common $P^1$ gene determining the P-positive blood. Although extremely rare as a cause of clinical symptoms, anti-**P** has been found following P-positive transfusions[12, 13] and has been reported as the cause of a fatal transfusion reaction.[14] Tests for the **P** factor are not considered sufficiently reliable for routine medicolegal purposes.

### Lutheran (Lu)

The next blood group system to be reported was named Lutheran after the name of the donor whose blood sensitized a patient.[15] The antigen, $Lu^a$, was inherited as a dominant Mendelian character and was present in about 7 percent of the English people. The entire system was further expanded with the finding of anti-$Lu^b$ [16] in 1956. Thus, the genotype frequencies are:

$$Lu^aLu^a = \phantom{0}1 \text{ percent}$$
$$Lu^aLu^b = \phantom{0}7 \text{ percent}$$
$$Lu^bLu^b = 92 \text{ percent}$$

Despite the rare presence of either a suppressor or the extremely rare Lu(a−b−) type, the Lutheran system is useful in paternity situations, where, because of the 8 percent frequency of $Lu^a$ persons, first order exclusions are possible and valid. The Lutheran antigen may not be well developed in infants and therefore warrants precautions in testing children under one year of age.[17] In addition, the type of agglutination produced by anti-$Lu^a$ is not typical since many nonagglutinated cells can be seen.

The interest in this system lies in the reported linkage between the Lutheran blood group and the secretor genes.[18, 19]

### The Duffy System (Fy)

Another newly discovered blood group system was described in 1950[20] and named Duffy; the genes determining the agglutinogens were named $Fy^a$ and $Fy^b$.[21] The inheritance is that of a simple Mendelian dominant. Population study revealed that the frequency of the Duffy types in Caucasians was:

$$Fy(a+b-) = 20 \text{ percent}$$
$$Fy(a-b+) = 34 \text{ percent}$$
$$Fy(a+b+) = 46 \text{ percent}$$
$$Fy(a-b-) = 0.1 \text{ percent}$$

This relationship was disturbed by the finding that approximately 70 percent of Negroes are $Fy(a-b-)$,[22] leading to the conclusion that there exists another allele at the Duffy locus which is an amorph, indicated as $Fy$. The antibodies for this system work best with the use of antiglobulin serum; the reactions with enzyme treated red cells are irregular.

This system has been implicated in several hemolytic transfusion reactions[23,224] and occasionally in erythroblastosis fetalis.[25, 26]

It has acceptability in medicolegal work only as a first order exclusion due to the presence of $Fy(a-b-)$ people (designated as $Fy$). $Fy$ people are especially found amongst Negroes, where this phenotype has a frequency of 70 percent.

## Kidd System (Jk)

Another blood group system, shown to be independent of A-B-O, Rh-Hr, M-N, P, Kell, Lutheran and Duffy was described in 1951.[27] This antibody was found in a case of hemolytic disease of the newborn and was named after the infant's mother. The antigen it recognized was named $Jk^a$ and was present in about 75 percent of Caucasians. Anti-$Jk^b$ was found in 1953.[28] This permitted the study of the frequency of the Jk type and the inheritance of the factors.

$$Jk^aJk^a = 24.5 \text{ percent}$$
$$Jk^aJk^b = 52.7 \text{ percent}$$
$$Jk^bJk^b = 22.5 \text{ percent}$$

A rare finding is the person whose red blood cells fail to react with either anti-$Jk^a$ or anti-$Jk^b$ serum. These few individuals[29] (designated Jk) indicate the presence of a third allele at the Jk locus. The antiserums for the **Jk** factors are weak and quickly lose their reactivity. They are best used by a combination of enzyme and antiglobulin technics as described by Unger.[30] The usefulness of this blood group system is seriously limited by the need for careful, complicated, and repeated testing technics to obtain reproducible results. Only first order exclusions are possible because of the silent allele Jk.

## Diego (Di) System

A distinctly unusual blood group system was demonstrated as being the exclusive property of Mongoloids by its discoverer, Layrisse.[31, 32] Two alleles, Di[a] and Di[b] have been described.[33] The antigens of this system appear solely in the blood of Chinese, Japanese, and American Indians. Clinically and medicolegally the Diego blood group is not of great significance; however, it does provide an important anthropological marker.

## Other Blood Factors

Many other blood factors have been reported that are not related to the A-B-O, M-N-S, P, Lewis, Rh-Hr, Lutheran, Kell, Duffy, Diego or Kidd systems. Further study may eventually demonstrate that these factors may be related to previously described blood groups or that they may even be duplicate examples of other factors. Several probably represent independent blood groups and are of sufficient frequency to deserve attention.

Those of greatest interest occur with high frequency in the general population. These have been named Vel,[34] I,[35] Yt[a],[36] and Xg.[37] Of lesser frequency are a large number of blood factors that have been identified in only one or two families. These often carry the name of the person in whose blood the antibody was first found. The problem of identifying such "family factors" are great—not infrequently duplication exists. The thrill of finding such a "previously unidentified antibody" that specifically recognizes an unknown antigen is the fitting reward of an alert laboratory worker. It is of medicolegal interest that the finding of a low-frequency factor in the blood of a child and its alleged father may indicate a high probability of paternity. For such a conclusion the factor must be of such infrequency in the general population as to preclude coincidence as an explanation.

## MEDICOLEGAL APPLICATIONS

The several blood group systems described in this chapter are not recommended for routine medicolegal use. Nevertheless, in the hands of a few qualified experts who possess the necessary testing serum and the essential control cells, in addition to the familiarity with the genetic principles of each of the blood groups, findings that indicate exclusions may be submitted to the court as evidence. In contrast to the exclusions based on A-B-O, Rh-Hr, and M-N-S, which many courts consider decisive, results of blood test findings in these other blood group systems should be subject to careful judicial evaluation.

## REFERENCES

1. Coombs, R. R. A., Mourant, A. E., and Race, R. R.: In vivo isosensitization of red cells in babies with haemolytic disease. *Lancet, 1:*264, 1946.

2. Wiener, A. S., and Sonn-Gordon, E. B.: Réaction transfusionnelle hemolytique intra-groupe due a un hémagglutinogen jusqù ici non décrit. *Rev. Hémat., 2:*1, 1947.

3. Levine, P., Backer, M., Wigod, M., and Ponder, R.: A new human hereditary blood property (Cellano) present in 99.8% of all bloods. *Science, 109:*464, 1949.

4. Allen, F., and Lewis, S. J.: Kp^a (Penny), a new antigen in the Kell blood group system. *Vox Sanguinis, 2:*81, 1957.

5. Allen, F. H., Lewis, S. J., and Fudenberg, H.: Studies of anti-Kp^b, a new antibody in the Kell blood group system. *Vox Sanguinis, 3:*1, 1958.

6. Chown, B., Lewis, M., and Kaita, H.: A "new" Kell blood group phenotype. *Nature,* London, *180:*711, 1957.

7. Stroup, M., MacIlroy, M., Walker, R., and Aydelotte, J. V.: Evidence that Sutter belongs to the Kell blood group system. *Transfusion,* 5:309-314, 1965.

8. Landsteiner, K., and Levine, P.: Further observations on individual differences of human blood. *Proc. Soc. Exper. Biol. & Med., N. Y., 24:* 941, 1927.

9. Landsteiner, K., and Levine, P.: On the inheritance and racial distribution of agglutinable properties of human blood. *J. Immunol., 18:*87, 1930.

10. Sanger, R.: An association between the P and Jay systems of blood groups. *Nature,* London, *176:*1163, 1955.

11. Levine, P., Bobbitt, O. B., Waller, R. K., and Kuhmichel, A.: Iso-im-

munization by a new blood factor in tumor cells. *Proc. Soc. Exper. Biol. & Med., N. Y.,* 77:403, 1951.

12. Wiener, A. S., and Peters, H. R.: Hemolytic reaction following transfusions of blood of the homologous group, with 3 cases in which the same agglutinogen was responsible. *Ann. Int. Med.,* 13:2306, 1940.

13. Wiener, A. S.: Hemolytic transfusion reactions. III. Prevention, with special reference to the Rh and cross-match tests. *Amer J. Clin. Path.,* 12:302, 1942.

14. Moureau, P.: Les réactions post-transfusionelles. *Rev. belge. Sci. Med.,* 16: 258, 1945.

15. Callender, S. R., and Race, R. R.: A serological and genetical study of multiple antibodies formed in response to blood transfusions by a patient with lupus erythematosis diffusus. *Ann. Eugenics,* 13:102, 1946.

16. Cutbush, M., and Chanarin, I.: The expected blood-group antibody, anti-Lu[b]. *Nature,* London, 178:855, 1956.

17. Greenwalt, T. J., Sasaki, T., and Steane, E. A.: The Lutheran blood group: a progress report with observations on the development of the antigens and characteristics of the antibodies. *Transfusion,* 7:189-200, 1967.

18. Mohr, J.: A search for linkage between the Lutheran blood group and other hereditary characters. *Acta Path. & Microbiol. Scand.,* 28:207, 1951.

19. Sanger, R., and Race, R. R.: The Lutheran-secretor linkage in man: support for Mohr's findings. *Heredity,* 12:513, 1958.

20. Cutbush, M., Mollison, P. L., and Parkin, D. M.: A new human blood group. *Nature,* London, 165:188, 1950.

21. Itkin, E. W., Mourant, A. E., Pettenkofer, H. J., and Blumenthal, G.: Discovery of the expected hemagglutinin anti-Fy[b]. *Nature,* London, 168:1077, 1951.

22. Sanger, R., Race, R. R., and Jack, J.: The Duffy blood group of New York Negroes: the phenotype Fy(a–b–). *Brit. J. Haemat.,* 1:370, 1955.

23. Freiesleben, E.: Fatal hemolytic transfusion reaction due to anti-Fy[a] (Duffy). *Acta Path. & Microbiol. Scand.,* 29:283, 1951.

24. Hutcheson, J. B., Haber, J. M., and Kellner, A.: A hazard of repeated blood transfusions. Hemolytic reaction due to antibodies to the Duffy (Fy[a]) factor. *J.A.M.A.,* 149:724, 1952.

25. Baker, J. B., Grewar, A., Lewis, M., Ayukawa, H., and Chown, B.: Haemolytic disease of the new born due to anti-Duffy (Fy[a]). *Arch. Dis. Child.,* 31:298, 1956.

26. Greenwalt, T. J., Sasaki, T., and Gajewski, M.: Further examples of

hemolytic disease of the new born to anti-Duffy (anti-Fy$^a$). *Vox Sanguinis,* 4:138, 1959.

27. Allen, F. H., Diamond, L. K., and Niedziela, B.: A new blood group antigen. *Nature,* London, 167:482, 1951.

28. Plaut, G., Ikin, E. W., Mourant, A. E., Sanger, R., and Race, R. R.: A new blood group antibody, anti-Jk$^b$. *Nature,* London, 171:431, 1953.

29. Sussman, L. N., Solomon, R., and Grogan, S.: The Kidd minus-minus phenotype. *Transfusion,* 15:356-358, 1975.

30. Unger, L. J.: A method for detecting Rh$_0$ antibodies in extremely low titer. *J. Lab. & Clin. Med.,* 37:825, 1951.

31. Layrisse, M., Arends, T., and Dominguez Sisco, R.: Nuevo grupo sanguineo encontrado en descendientes de Indios. *Acta Medica Venezolana,* 3:132, 1955.

32. Levine, P., Robinson, E. A., Layrisse, M., Arends, T., and Dominguez Sisco, R.: The Diego blood factor. *Nature,* London, 177:40, 1956.

33. Thompson, P. R., Childers, D. M., and Hatcher, D. E.: Anti-Di$^b$—First and second examples. *Vox Sanguinis,* 13:314, 1967.

34. Sussman, L. N., and Miller, E. B.: Un nouveau facteur sanguin "Vel." *Rev. Hémat.,* 7:368, 1952.

35. Wiener, A. S., Unger, L. J., Cohen, L., and Feldman, J.: Type-specific cold auto-antibodies as a cause of acquired hemolytic anemia and hemolytic transfusion reactions: biologic test with bovine red cells. *Ann. Int. Med.,* 44:221, 1956.

36. Eaton, B. R., Morton, J. A., Pickles, M. M., and White, K. E.: A new antibody anti-Yt$^a$ characterizing a blood group of high incidence. *Brit. J. Haemat.,* 2:333, 1956.

37. Mann, J. D., Cahan, A., Gelb, A. G., Fisher, N., Hamper, J., Tippett, P., Sanger, R. and Race, R. R.: A sex linked blood group. *Lancet,* 1:8-10, 1962.

CHAPTER SIX

# SERUM PROTEINS AND ERYTHROCYTE ENZYMES

H. F. POLESKY AND DALE DYKES

## PRINCIPLES

IN THE PREVIOUS EDITION of this book a chapter entitled "A Preview of the Future in Blood Grouping Tests" was included. The material to follow shows that the future referred to in 1968 is now.

The utilization of systems other than red cell antigen polymorphisms in establishing nonpaternity is based on a history of careful investigative work. The demonstration by Pauling et al.,[1] that sickle-cell disease was caused by an easily distinguishable, abnormal hemoglobin, which is also identified in individuals with sickle trait, initiated these investigations. Oliver Smithies'[2] development of starch gel electrophoresis and his subsequent studies of the haptoglobin polymorphism[3, 4] opened the way for the discovery of numerous new systems.

As with various blood group antigens certain generalizations apply to all systems. Prior to using one of these markers to exclude paternity one must be certain there is firm evidence with adequate family studies to show that the characteristic follows the expected inheritance pattern. Extreme caution must be used in interpreting results where the putative father is apparently homozygous for a characteristic absent in the child, i.e. exclusion of the second class. Silent alleles, deletions, and failure to be developed at an early age all must be considered in evaluating test results.

The population from which the sample is drawn is important in selecting which tests to use. Some systems, like hemoglobin, show such little variation in one population (whites) as to be useless, while in another group they may be quite polymorphic (sickle hemoglobin in 8-11% of blacks).[5]

Another important consideration before employing tests is knowledge that the protein or enzyme is stable under the conditions which will be used to store specimens prior to testing.

## TECHNIQUES AND APPLICATIONS
### Erythrocyte Enzymes

Over a dozen enzyme systems with genetic variants have been described since Hopkinson demonstrated that hemolysates of human erythrocytes contained a polymorphic enzyme system, red cell acid phosphatase (acP).[6] The basic method for studying these systems is to separate their isoenzymes by starch gel electrophoresis. The various bands produced are then visualized on the gel by their reaction with a substrate specific for the system under study.

### Sample Collection and Preparation

Samples for erythrocyte enzyme tests are best collected in tubes containing ACD or Alsevers solution. The presence of dextrose helps maintain several enzymes.[7] Erythrocytes from clots and other anticoagulants can be used, but results are less satisfactory in those systems in which the amount of enzyme activity drops as the cells age. We have had good results with most systems if hemolysates are prepared from clots within a week after drawing. Clots should be refrigerated until processing can be done. We also recommend that samples to be mailed to another laboratory for testing be refrigerated prior to shipping. Precooled samples placed in styrofoam mailers without ice, etc. are satisfactory for testing most systems.

Hemolysates are prepared from erythrocytes washed at least four times with several volumes of saline. An equal volume of distilled water is added to the well washed packed cells which are hemolyzed by repeated freezing and thawing. Hemolysates can also be prepared by sonication of the washed, packed cells. A few drops of digitonin in saline (5 mg/ml) added to the specimen prior to centrifugation at 1880 G will provide a stroma free hemolysate. If samples cannot be run on the day the hemolysate is prepared, they can be stored frozen for several months to several years depending on the systems to be used. For longer term frozen storage of hemolysates one drop of 0.02 M 2-mercaptoethanol should be added to preserve ADA and acP.[8]

## Electrophoretic Method

The conditions of the electrophoretic run vary with different enzyme systems. One of the routine methods in the author's laboratory is as follows:

1. Prepare pH 5.9 phosphate (0.245M $NaH_2PO_4$) citrate (0.15M $Na_3C_6H_5O_72H_2O$) *bridge buffer.*
2. A 1:60 dilution of the bridge buffer is used as the *gel buffer.*
3. 11-13g/dl of hydrolyzed starch (exact amount varies from lot to lot) is added to 160 ml of the gel buffer in a large flask.
4. 340 ml of gel buffer is heated to 103°C.
5. The heated gel buffer is added to the starch-buffer mixture (Step 3).
6. While hot the 500 ml of starch is degassed under gentle vacuum.
7. Pour the degassed mixture into an 18 cm. × 32 cm. × 0.6 cm. form (see Figure 6-1).
8. Cover the form with a prewarmed glass plate and allow starch to solidify at room temperature.

Hemolysates are used to saturate 10 mm by 3 mm pieces of thick filter paper which are then inserted in the solid gel 10 cms from the cathodal end. By careful spacing, eight samples can be run on each gel.

Gels are electrophoresed in a horizontal position at 4°C for seventeen hours. Voltage (7.5 V/cm) is applied using a Health Kit Model IP-17 power supply attached to the 500 ml buffer chambers which contain the undiluted bridge buffer. Under these discontinuous conditions, hemoglobin should migrate cathodally 6 cm from the origin.

Utilizing the system described, one electrophoretic run makes it possible to study four enzyme systems if the gel slab is carefully sliced and correctly divided (see Fig. 6-1). AK, 6-PGD, and

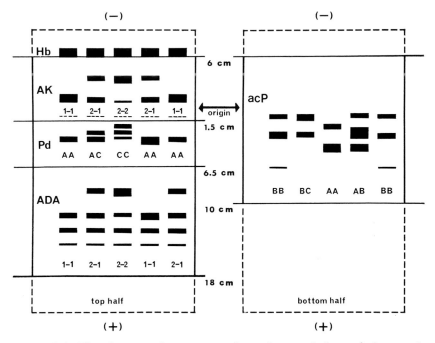

Figure 6-1. This diagram demonstrates how the two halves of the starch gel are cut to phenotype four enzyme systems. Distances given are from the point of origin and apply to gels run under the conditions described in the text. The band patterns of common phenotypes for each system are shown.

ADA are localized in sections of one-half the gel and are stained using the technics of Brinkmann[9] modified by increasing the quantities of recommended reagents by 25 percent. The remaining one half of the gel is used for phenotyping acid phosphatase. Of these four enzymes, only acid phosphatase is polymorphic enough to be routinely discriminating. The others, though not very polymorphic, have been useful in determining exclusions and in calculating paternity indexes.

### Useful Systems

In the author's laboratory, in addition to the systems mentioned above, tests for $PGM_1$ and esterase D are routine. Others[10] have used GPT, but the authors have had difficulty getting re-

TABLE 6-I

| RBC Enzymes (Synonyms) | Function | Common Alleles | Rare Alleles |
|---|---|---|---|
| *Adenosine Deaminase*<br>ADA<br>E.C.   3.5.4.4. | Catalyzes deamination of adenosine to inosine | $ADA^1$, $ADA^2$ | $ADA^3$ $ADA^4$, $ADA^5$ |
| *Adenylate Kinase*<br>AK<br>Myokinase<br>AMP phosphotransferase;<br>E.C.   2.7.4.3. | Catalyzes $2ADP \rightleftharpoons ATP + AMP$ | $AK^1$, $AK^2$ | $AK^3$, $AK^4$, $AK^5$ |
| *6-Phosphogluconate Dehydrogenase*<br>6-PGD<br>D-glucose-1-phosphate phosphotransferase;<br>E.C.   1.1.1.44. | Catalyzes oxidative decarboxylation of 6PG to R5P | $PGD^A$, $PGD^C$ | $PGD^F$, $PGD^H$, $PGD^R$, $PGD^S$, $PGD^{Thai}$, $PGD^{Elco}$ |
| *Phosphoglucomutase*<br>PGM<br>$\alpha$-D-glucose-1, 6 diphosphate:<br>$\alpha$-D-glucose-1-phosphate phosphotransferase;<br>E.C.   2.7.5.1. | Catalyzes $G\text{-}I\text{-}P \rightleftharpoons G\text{-}6\text{-}P$ | $PGM_1^1$, $PGM_1^2$ | $PGM_1^3$, $PGM_1^4$,<br><br>$PGM_1^5$, $PGM_1^6$,<br><br>$PGM_1^7$, $PGM_1^8$ |
| *Acid Phosphatase*<br>acP | Phosphotrans-ferase activity | $p^A$, $p^B$, $p^C$ | $p^R$, $p^D$, $p^{EB}$ |
| *Glutamic-Pyruvic Transaminase*<br>GPT<br>Alanine amino-transferase:<br>E.C.   2.6.1.2. | Reversible interconversion of 1-alanine and $\alpha$-ketogluterate to 1-glutamate and pyruvate | $Gpt^1$, $Gpt^2$ | $Gpt^3$, $Gpt^4$, $Gpt^5$, $Gpt^6$, $Gpt^7$ |
| *Esterase D* | Esterase activity | $EsD^1$, $EsD^2$ | $EsD^3$ |

Table 6-I (cont.)

| Quantitative Variants | Probability of Obtaining an Exclusion Population | | References Methods | References Genetics and Population Studies | References Use in Paternity Testing |
| --- | --- | --- | --- | --- | --- |
| | White | Black | | | |
| ADA$^O$ | 0.0452 | 0.0192 | 9, 30, 31 | 8, 32, 33, 34, 35 | 36 |
| AK$^O$ | 0.0429 | 0.0066 | 9, 31, 37 38, 39 | 40, 41 | |
| Ilford, Newman, Whitechapel, Dalston | 0.0229 | 0.0326 | 9, 39, 42, 43 | 44, 45, 46, 47, 48 | |
| PGM$_1^{1R}$ | 0.1421 | 0.1186 | 31, 39, 49 | 50, 51 | 52, 53 |
| P$^O$ | 0.2508 | 0.1544 | 31, 49, 54, 55, 56 | 6, 57, 58, 59 60 | 61, 62 |
| Gpt$^{1M}$, Gpt$^O$ | 0.1875 | 0.1285 | 39, 63, 64 | 10, 65, 66 | |
| | 0.0806 | 0.0806 | 67, 68 | 69, 70 | |

producible results. Glucose-6-phosphate dehydrogenase (G-6-PD) is another system that is used on occasion. This enzyme is controlled by an X-linked gene and therefore is only useful in evaluating nonpaternity of female children.[11]

Rather than present a detailed description of each enzyme system, pertinent facts have been summarized in Table 6-I. References to papers on methodology, genetic variants, and the application of the given system in paternity testing are included in the table.

## Pitfalls

It should be noted that amorphs and/or alleles with low activity have been reported in most enzyme systems. Thus, it may be necessary to do quantitative assays of enzyme levels when there is an uncorroborated exclusion of the second class. Such assays should always include appropriate controls, i.e. known homozygotes and heterozygotes collected and stored for similar lengths of time. Other studies that can be useful in differentiating gene products include evaluation of Km values with different substrates, measurements of pH optimums, determination of thermostability, and the effects of various inhibitors.

## Application to Paternity Testing

Table 6-I includes data on the probability of obtaining an exclusion of paternity if the only markers tested for were those in the system listed. The differences in usefulness between whites and blacks depends on the relative frequency of the genes in each population. Table 6-II shows phenotype frequencies for several enzyme systems. From this information, one can see why PGM$_1$ can be useful in testing falsely accused individuals from either a white or black population. PGM$_2$, on the other hand, would be of relatively little use in either group.

Table 6-III summarizes the exclusions we have observed in a series of 281 white families using five enzymes systems. Fifty-two of the 281 putative fathers were excluded on the basis of all tests (red cell antigens, serum proteins and red cell enzymes). First class exclusions based on enzyme systems totalled nineteen

TABLE 6-II

POPULATION DATA—ERYTHROCYTE ENZYMES

| | Phenotype Frequency (%) | | | |
|---|---|---|---|---|
| System | 1-1 | 2-1 | 2-2 | Other |
| Phosphoglucomutase | | | | |
| PGM₁ | | | | |
| White | 55.9 | 35.1 | 7.9 | 1.1 |
| Black | 59.1 | 35.1 | 3.9 | 1.9 |
| PGM₂ | | | | |
| White | 98.5 | 0.5 | 0 | 1.0 |
| Black | 99.4 | 0 | 0 | 0.6 |
| Adenylate kinase | | | | |
| White | 97.3 | 2.7 | 0 | 0 |
| Black | 100 | 0 | 0 | 0 |
| Adenosine deaminase | | | | |
| White | 88.1 | 11.9 | 0 | 0 |
| Black | 97.2 | 2.8 | 0 | 0 |

\* Data from studies on 180 white and 180 black individuals residing in Philadelphia, Pennsylvania.[71]

or 37.3 percent of the falsely accused males. This figure (37.3%) is quite close to the expected (cumulative P = 0.4261) chance of obtaining an exclusion with these systems when testing a white population.

## Serum Proteins

During the last forty years numerous protein species have been isolated and characterized by physical, chemical, and other techniques.[12] Specific functions and changes in disease states have

TABLE 6-III

ENZYME EXCLUSIONS FOUND IN 281 PATERNITY CASES

| Class of Exclusion | AK | Enzyme System | | | | Total Number |
|---|---|---|---|---|---|---|
| | | ADA | PGD | acP | PGM₁ | |
| 1 | 3 | 1 | 0 | 12 | 3 | 19 |
| 2 | 1 | 0 | 0 | 3 | 1 | 5 |
| Total observed | 4 | 1 | 0 | 15 | 4 | 24 |
| Total expected\* | 2.19 | 2.30 | 1.17 | 12.8 | 7.25 | 21.7\*\* |

\* In 52 falsely accused males.
\*\* Based on cumulative P = 0.4261.

been defined for many but not all of these proteins. Most proteins are polymorphic and under genetic control.

## Sample Collection and Preservation

Serum from freshly clotted samples is ideal for tests to determine protein phenotypes. Plasma can also be used in many systems. Although refrigeration is recommended for short term and freezing for long term storage of specimens, the authors have obtained good results on samples left on the cells for many weeks and/or stored under less than ideal conditions. The stability of each system, changes produced by storage and the effects of contamination must be considered in interpreting results.

## Acrylamide Gel Electrophoresis

Separation of the closely related variants within a given species of protein usually requires a combination of electrophoresis and a medium with some molecular sieving properties.[13, 14] In the author's laboratory polyacrylamide gels are used for these studies. The method is as follows:

1. Prepare a pH 8.29 TEB buffer-tris (0.9M), EDTA (0.0025M Na$_2$EDTA), borate (0.08M H$_3$BO$_3$).
2. In one liter of the TEB buffer dissolve 70 gms. of Cyanogum 41 (EC Apparatus Company, St. Petersburg, Florida).
3. Filter the acrylamide solution three times to remove debris and undissolved cyanogum.
4. To initiate polymerization add 0.2 gms. of ammonium persulfate and 0.25 ml. of TMED (N,N,N',N'-tetramethylene diamine) to 250 ml. of the 7.0 g/dl acrylamide.
5. After mixing to dissolve the ammonium persulfate the solution (Step 4) is added to a gel form taking care to avoid trapping air (see Figure 6-2).

The gel form is left horizontal for at least thirty minutes to insure complete polymerization. Excess acrylamide above the sample slot former is removed and the form placed upright. The buffer chambers are filled with cold (4°C) buffer. The slot former is removed and the refrigerant circulation through the jacket surrounding the gel is started. Prior to adding samples, a thirty-

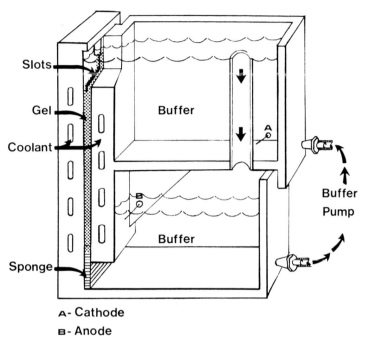

Slots

Gel

Coolant

Buffer

A

Buffer
Pump

B

Buffer

Sponge

A- Cathode

B- Anode

Figure 6-2. This diagram shows a cutaway side view of the electrophoresis apparatus used to run acrylamide gel slabs. The gels shown in Figures 6-3 and 6-4 were prepared by this method.[15] Note the coolant plates to prevent heating during the run and the circulation of buffer between lower and upper chambers to minimize electrolytic changes.

minute prerun at 60 ma is done to equilibrate the gel and buffer phases. This improves resolution. With the power off, 20 $\mu$l of serum is added to each sample slot. After the samples have evenly layered in the slots the current is again applied at 60 ma for thirty minutes. A pump for circulating the buffer between upper and lower chambers is started and the power supply adjusted to deliver 250 volts (100-150 ma). The run is continued for three-and-one-half hours. After disconnecting the power, the gel slab is removed and placed in a dish of boiling 5% acetic acid for five to fifteen minutes to fix the protein bands. This prevents migration during staining. Gel slabs are placed in 0.7 g/dl amido black dissolved in methyl alcohol (5 parts), glacial acetic acid (½ part), water (5 parts) overnight. They are then destaining

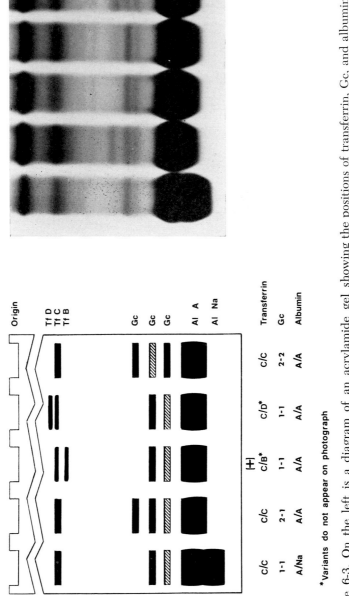

Figure 6-3. On the left is a diagram of an acrylamide gel showing the positions of transferrin, Gc, and albumin bands. On the right is a photo of a gel with the same albumin and Gc phenotypes. The sample with Albumin Naskapi ($Al^A/Al^{Na}$) is from an Ojibwa Indian. Note that staining intensity (as indicated by cross-hatching) is used to determine Gc phenotype.

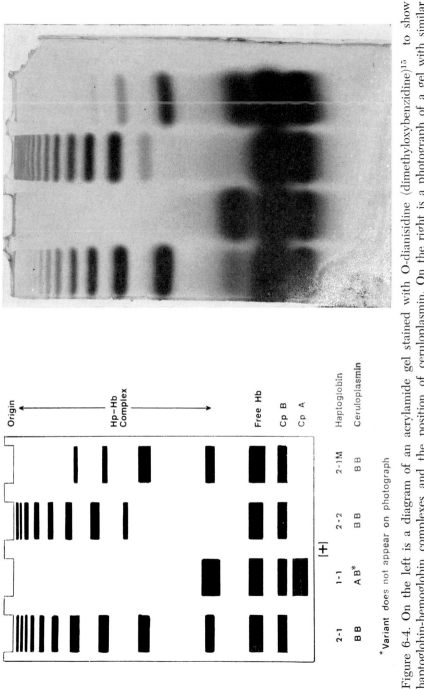

Figure 6-4. On the left is a diagram of an acrylamide gel stained with O-dianisidine (dimethyloxybenzidine)[15] to show haptoglobin-hemoglobin complexes and the position of ceruloplasmin. On the right is a photograph of a gel with similar haptoglobin phenotypes. The last slot shows a 2-1 mod. This variant of haptoglobin occurs in blacks and is characterized by a lower capacity to bind hemoglobin and fewer bands in the cathodal region.

using the solvent described for the amido black. To speed up this process an electrophoretic destainer can be used. Typing of proteins such as transferrin and albumin depend on the position of the various bands (Fig. 6-3). In evaluating other proteins, such as Gc, one has to consider staining intensity as well as position to determine the phenotype.

Two useful proteins, haptoglobin and ceruloplasmin, are typed by observing the position of bands reacting with specific substrates. Since heat can destroy enzyme activity, the acetic acid step and staining procedure are changed when studying these systems[15] (Fig. 6-4).

### Immunologic Methods

Another approach to the study of polymorphic proteins utilizes immunoelectrophoresis. Hirschfeld[16] discovered the Gc polymorphism by observing the position of the precipitin arcs following electrophoresis. This method depends on the availability of well characterized antisera to the specific protein. The authors have achieved only limited success with this technic.

Immunodiffusion technics have been used to define several low-density β-lipoprotein systems.[17–19] These tests have several pitfalls not the least of which is the lack of stability of the antigen.

Passive hemagglutination inhibition tests are used to determine the Gm (the Genetic Marker or Gamma globulin system) factors of an individual. This highly informative system results from peptide variations in the "constant" portion of the heavy chains of IgG.[20] Similar technics are also used in tests for the Inv markers found on the kappa light chains of all Ig molecules, and the Am marker of the alpha chains.

GM: To determine Gm, incomplete Rh antibodies (IgG) that have been characterized for their Gm markers are coated onto group O, Rh-positive erythrocytes. These coated cells serve as indicators in an inhibition system consisting of the unknown serum and antibody against a specific Gm factor. If the unknown lacks the particular Gm factor, the coated red cells are agglutinated by the antibody (anti-Gm). If the specific factor is present in the unknown, hemagglutination is inhibited. Though this sys-

TABLE 6-IV

NOMENCLATURE FOR IMMUNOGLOBULIN MARKERS

| Chain Type | Designation Alphameric | Numeric |
|---|---|---|
| IgG₁ .................................. Glm | a | 1 |
| | x | 2 |
| | f | 3 |
| | z | 17 |
| IgG₂ .................................. G2m | n | 23 |
| IgG₃ .................................. G3m | b0 | 11 |
| | b1 | 5 |
| | b3 | 13 |
| | b4 | 14 |
| | b5 | 10 |
| | c3 | 6 |
| | c5 | 24 |
| | g | 21 |
| | s | 15 |
| | t | 16 |
| | u | 26 |
| | v | 27 |
| IgA₂ .................................. A2m | 1 | 1 |
| | 2 | 2 |
| Kappa chains (Formerly Inv) .............. Km | 1 | 1 |
| | 2 (a) | 2 |
| | 3 (b) | 3 |

TABLE 6-V

FREQUENCY

| Gene Complex | White | Frequency Black | Japanese | Chinese |
|---|---|---|---|---|
| fb¹b⁵ ...................... | .69 | 0 | 0 | 0 |
| azg ....................... | .20 | 0 | .47 | .23 |
| azxg ...................... | .10 | 0 | .17 | .09 |
| azb¹b⁵ ..................... | <.01 | .55 | <.01 | <.01 |
| azb¹c³c⁵ .................... | <.01 | .25 | 0 | 0 |
| azb⁵s ...................... | 0 | .11 | 0 | 0 |
| azb¹b⁵c³ ................... | 0 | .08 | 0 | 0 |
| azb⁵st ..................... | <.01 | 0 | .28 | .06 |
| afb¹b⁵ ..................... | 0 | 0 | .08 | .62 |

Table 6-VI

Summary of Serum Protein Systems

| Serum Proteins (Synonyms) | Function | Common Alleles | Rare Alleles |
|---|---|---|---|
| *Gc–Globulin* Group–Specific Components Gc Components Gc Factor | Unknown | $Gc^1$, $Gc^2$ | 10+ variants |
| *Ceruloplasmin* | Cooper binding glycoprotein, ferro-oxidase activity | $Cp^A$, $Cp^B$ | $Cp^C$, $Cp^{NH}$, $Cp^{Bpt}$, $Cp^{Gal}$, $Cp^{Thai}$, $Cp^{Nia}$, $Cp^{1F}$, Cayopa, Yanomama |
| *Haptoglobin* Seromucoid *a2* | Binding of free Hb in plasma | $Hp^1$, $Hp^2$ | $Hp^J$, $Hp^{1D}$, $Hp^{1B}$, $Hp^L$, $Hp^P$, $Hp^H$ |
| *Transferrin* Siderophilin, $\beta_1$ S-globulin, $\beta_1$ Metal combining globulin | Iron-binding and iron transport in plasma | $Tf^C$, $Tf^{D1}$ | 17+ variants |
| *C3 Component* $\beta_1$ C-globulin C3 complement | Key protein in complement sequence. | S, F | 10+ variants |
| *Gm* | Unknown | 20 Factors, 9 major haplo types | Gm (f;g), deletions and cross overs reported |
| *Inv* *Km* | Unknown | Inv (1,2) Inv (3) | Inv (1,-2) |

Table 6-VI (cont.)

Summary of Serum Protein Systems

| Quantitative Variants | Probability of Obtaining an Exclusion Population White | Black | References Methods | References Genetics and Population Studies | References Use in Paternity Testing |
|---|---|---|---|---|---|
| Gc$^O$ | 0.1554 | 0.0819 | 15, 72, 73, 74, 75 | 76, 77, 78, 79 | 80, 81 |
| | 0.0059 | 0.0510 | 15, 82, 83, 84 | 78, 85, 86, 87 88 | |
| Hp$^{Ca}$, Hp$^{2M}$, Hp$^{Haw}$, Hp$^{Trans}$, Hp$^O$ | 0.1806 | 0.1555 | 15 | 78, 89, 90, 91 92 | 93 |
| | 0.0059 | 0.0499 | 15, 94 | 78, 95 | |
| C3$^O$ | 0.1423 | 0.0623 | 96 | 97, 98, 99, 100 | 101 |
| | 0.2253 | 0.2065 | 21, 102 | 22, 23, 25, 26, 27, 103, 104, 105 | 106, 107, 108 |
| | 0.0799 | 0.1739 | 21 | 22, 103 | |

tem depends on the availability of scarce reagents (appropriate anti-Rh coats and anti-Gm) only minimal quantities are required if a microtiter system is utilized. Detailed descriptions of the method can be found in *Paternity Testing* (edited by Polesky).[21]

If one uses Gm in paternity tests, certain pitfalls must be kept in mind. Deletions, crossing over, failure to develop before three months of age and disease state (myeloma, immune deficiency) are potential sources of error in interpretation.[22, 23] Another source of problems is the confusion that has resulted from the use of two nomenclatures in publications on Gm. Certain factors have acquired multiple designations which recently have been standardized by a WHO workshop[24] (see Table 6-IV).

## Exclusion of Paternity without a Maternal Sample

Table 6-V shows the distribution of the Gm gene complexes (haplotypes) in four populations.[25–27] It should be noted that in each group at least three haplotypes occur with a frequency of 9 percent or more. Thus, it is possible to encounter a child who has two haplotypes absent in the accused man. For example:

| | |
|---|---|
| Child | azxg/fb¹b⁵ |
| Putative father | azg/azg. |

Data such as this can establish nonpaternity without a maternal sample. A similar situation occurs when an O male is accused of fathering an AB child or in the acP erythrocyte enzyme system when the child is $P^AP^A$ and the accused man $P^BP^C$.

## Use of Protein Systems

Rather than give a detailed description of each system, Table 6-VI summarizes key data about some of the useful proteins. References to methods, variants, and use in paternity tests are included for each system.

As with erythrocyte enzymes the phenotypic distribution and thus the usefulness of a protein varies depending on the population from which the sample is drawn. Table 6-VII illustrates the variability of several markers in white, black and American Indian (Ojibwa) populations the authors have studied. From

TABLE 6-VII

POPULATION DATA—PROTEINS

| System | Phenotype Frequency (%) | | | | |
|---|---|---|---|---|---|
| Transferrin | CC | CD | DD | | |
| White[*] | 99.5 | 0.5 | 0 | | |
| Black[*] | 93.5 | 6.0 | 0.5 | | |
| Haptoglobin | 1-1 | 2-1 | 2-2 | 21 Mod | 0-0 |
| White | 15.8 | 48.8 | 35.3 | 0 | 0 |
| Black | 32.4 | 35.9 | 24.1 | 5.9 | 1.8 |
| Ojibwa[**] | 17.4 | 48.3 | 34.3 | 0 | 0 |
| Gc | 1-1 | 2-1 | 2-2 | Other | |
| White | 48.0 | 46.0 | 6.0 | 0 | |
| Black | 73.7 | 23.4 | 2.4 | 0.5 | |
| Ojibwa | 55.4 | 30.5 | 4.3 | 9.8 | |
| Albumin | $Al^A Al^A$ | $Al^A Al^{Na}$ | $Al^{Na} Al^{Na}$ | | |
| White | 100 | 0 | 0 | | |
| Black | 100 | 0 | 0 | | |
| Ojibwa | 96 | 3.5 | 0.5 | | |

[*] Data from studies on 180 white and 180 black individuals residing in Philadelphia, Pennsylvania.[71]

[**] Data from 490 residents on Leech Lake Reservation.[109]

the data presented it should be clear that specifically testing for albumin will be of no value in trying to establish non paternity in Philadelphia. If a paternity case involves an Ojibwa Indian or another individual from a population in which albumin is polymorphic, then the test may help discriminate among random individuals in that population. If one of the rare variants such as Albumin Gainseville, etc.[28] is found in both the putative father and child, this would be presumptive evidence of paternity. Such information is useful when the putative father is compared to random individuals but must be interpreted with caution if dealing with a related male.

## Application of Proteins to Paternity Testing

Table 6-VIII shows the exclusions observed by including four serum protein systems in routine tests for establishing nonpaternity. This data is from the same 281 white families included in Table 6-III. The four systems used have a cumulative P = 0.316

TABLE 6-VIII

PROTEIN EXCLUSIONS FOUND IN 281 PATERNITY CASES

| *Class of Exclusion* | *Hp* | *Protein System* | | *Cp* | *Total Number* |
|:---:|:---:|:---:|:---:|:---:|:---:|
| | | *Gc* | *Tf* | | |
| 1 ................... | 5 | 5 | 1 | 0 | 11 |
| 2 ................... | 3 | 0 | 0 | 0 | 3 |
| Total observed ............. | 8 | 5 | 1 | 0 | 14 |
| Total expected* ........... | 9.2 | 7.9 | 0.30 | 0.30 | 16** |

　* In 52 falsely accused males.
　** Based on cumulative P = 0.316.

$$= 1 - (1 - 0.1806)(1 - 0.1554)(1 - 0.0059)(1 - 0.0059)^{29}$$ and should have excluded sixteen of the falsely accused males. As seen in Table 6-VIII, the authors observed eleven first-class and three second-class exclusions with these tests.

If only ABO, Rh, MNSs had been used in testing the 281 families, the authors would have been able to exclude 57.8 percent of the falsely accused males. With only red cell enzymes (acP, $PGM_1$, ADA, AK, 6-PD) and serum protein (Hp, Gc, Cp, Tf) testing, 60.4 percent could be excluded. However, combining all the tests one could expect to correctly identify 83.3 percent of falsely accused males. In addition to improving the rate of exclusion, erythrocyte enzymes and serum proteins have been helpful in providing corroborative evidence in exclusions of the second class and in determining paternity indexes. The following three cases illustrate the usefulness of these systems in paternity disputes.

*CASE 1*

| | *Blood Group* | *$Rh_o(D)$* | *$rh'(C)$* | *$rh''(E)$* | *$hr'(c)$* | *$hr''(e)$* | *M* | *N* | *S* | *s* | *K* | *k* | *$Inv(1)$* | *acP* |
|---|---|---|---|---|---|---|---|---|---|---|---|---|---|---|
| Alleged Father | $A_1$ | − | − | − | + | + | − | + | − | + | − | + | − | BB |
| Mother | $A_1$ | + | + | + | + | + | + | + | + | + | − | + | − | AB |
| Child | O | + | + | − | − | + | + | + | + | + | − | + | + | AA |

Additional tests performed in the author's laboratory included studies on the serum protein polymorphisms, transferrin, haptoglobin, albumin, Gc protein, ceruloplasmin and Gm, the red cell enzyme systems, PGM-1, PGM-2, ADA, AKA, 6-PGD. None of the above tests were informative in this case.

INTERPRETATION:

Exclusion of paternity on Rh, acid phosphatase and Inv.

The exclusion is based on finding that the Inv(1) factor in the child is absent in both the putative father and mother. In order for a child to inherit Inv(1), one of the parents must possess the gene for this characteristic. This exclusion is corroborated by findings in the Rh system. The alleged father is of the phenotype rhrh and the child of the phenotype $Rh_1Rh_1$. Any child of this man should therefore receive the *r* gene and since this child did not, this is evidence of nonpaternity. The finding that the alleged father is of the acid phosphatase phenotype BB and the child lacks evidence of the *B* gene is further evidence of nonpaternity.

Note: The Inv(1) exclusion is of the first order while those in the Rh and acP systems are of the second class.

| CASE 2 | *Blood Group* | *Rh$_o$(D)* | *rh'(C)* | *rh"(E)* | *hr'(c)* | *hr"(e)* | *M* | *N* | *S* | *s* | *K* | *k* | *EsD* | *Gm* |
|---|---|---|---|---|---|---|---|---|---|---|---|---|---|---|
| Alleged Father | A | + | − | + | + | + | − | + | − | + | − | + | 1-1 | azfb¹b⁵ |
| Mother | B | + | + | + | + | + | + | + | + | + | − | + | 1-1 | azb¹b⁵ |
| Child | B | + | − | + | + | + | + | + | + | + | − | + | 2-1 | azb¹b⁵c³c⁵ |

Additional tests performed in the author's laboratory included studies on the serum protein polymorphisms transferrin, haptoglobin, albumin, Gc protein, ceruloplasmin, and Inv; the red cell enzyme systems, acid phosphatase, PGM-1, PGM-2, ADA, AKA, 6-PGD. None of the above tests were informative in this case.

INTERPRETATION:

Exclusion of paternity on esterase D and Gm.

At least one parent of an EsD 2-1 child must have the gene for *EsD2*. This gene is absent in both the mother and alleged father, thus establishing nonpaternity. This is confirmed by finding that Gm C³ and C⁵ in the child is absent in the mother and accused male. The most probable Gm genotypes are as follows:

$$\begin{array}{ll}
\text{Alleged Father} & \text{azb}^1\text{b}^5/\text{fb}^1\text{b}^5 \\
\text{Mother} & \text{azb}^1\text{b}^5/\text{azb}^1\text{b}^5 \\
\text{Child} & \text{azb}^1\text{b}^5\text{c}^3\text{c}^5/\text{azb}^1\text{b}^5
\end{array}$$

NOTE: In both systems the exclusions are of the first order.

*CASE 3*

| | Blood Group | $Rh_o(D)$ | $rh'(C)$ | $rh^{1w}(C^w)$ | $rh''(E)$ | $hr'(c)$ | $hr''(e)$ | M | N | S | s | K | k | Hp |
|---|---|---|---|---|---|---|---|---|---|---|---|---|---|---|
| Alleged Father | O | + | + | − | − | − | + | + | + | + | + | − | + | 1-1 |
| Mother | A | + | + | − | − | + | + | + | + | + | + | − | + | 1-1 |
| Child | A | + | + | − | − | + | + | + | − | − | + | − | + | 2-1 |

Additional tests performed in the author's laboratory included studies on the serum protein polymorphisms, transferrin, albumin, Gc protein, ceruloplasmin, Gm and Inv; the red cell enzyme systems, acid phosphatase, PGM-1, PGM-2, ADA, AKA, 6-PGD. None of the above tests were informative in this case.

INTERPRETATION:

Exclusion of paternity on haptoglobin.

The exclusion in this case is based on finding a 2-1 haptoglobin in the child from a supposed 1-1 × 1-1 mating. The absence of the *Hp2* gene in both the mother and alleged father establishes a first order exclusion of paternity.

### REFERENCES

1. Pauling, L., Itano, H. A., Singer, S. J., and Wells, I. C.: Sickle cell anemia, a molecular disease. *Science, 110:*543-548, 1949.
2. Smithies, O.: Zone electrophoresis in starch gels: group variations in serum proteins of normal human adults. *Biochem. J., 61:*641, 1955.
3. Smithies, O., and Walker, N. F.: Notation for serum protein groups and the genes controlling their inheritance. *Nature, 178:*694-695, 1956.
4. Smithies, O., Connell, G. E., and Dixon, G. H.: Inheritance of haptoglobin subtypes. *Am. J. Hum. Genet., 14:*14-21, 1962.
5. Binder, R. A., and Jones, S. R.: Prevalence and awareness of sickle cell hemoglobins in a military population. *J.A.M.A., 214:*909-911, 1970.
6. Hopkinson, D. A., Spencer, N., and Harris, H.: Red cell acid phos-

phatase variants: a new human polymorphism. *Nature, 199*:969, 1963.

7. Brewer, G. J.: *Introduction to Isozyme Techniques.* New York, Academic Press, 1970, pp. 53-55.

8. Shinoda, T.: Polymorphism of red cell adenosine deaminase in the Japanese population. *Japan J. Genetics, 45*:147-152, 1970.

9. Brinkmann, B., and Thoma, G.: Simultaneous electrophoresis of three isoenzyme polymorphisms; 6 phosphogluconate dehydrogenase (6-PGD), adenosine deaminase (ADA), adenylate kinase (AK). *Vox Sang., 21*:93, 1971.

10. Chen, S-H., Giblett, E. R., and Anderson, J. E.: Genetics of glutamic-pyruvic transaminase: its inheritance, common and rare alleles, population distribution and differences in catalytic activity. *Ann. Hum. Genet., 35*:401, 1972.

11. Gross, R. T., Hurwitz, R. R., and Marks, P. A.: An hereditary enzymatic defect in erythrocyte metabolism: G-6-PD deficiency. *J. Clin. Invest., 37*:1176, 1958.

12. Schultze, H. E., and Heremans, J. F.: *Molecular Biology of Human Proteins.* Amsterdam, Elsevier, 1966, vol. 1.

13. Smithies, O.: "Zone Electrophoresis in Starch Gels and Its Application to Studies of Serum Protein," in Anfinsen, C. B. et al. (eds.), *Advances in Protein Chemistry.* New York, Academic Press, 1959, vol. 14, p. 65.

14. Raymond, S.: Acrylamide gel electrophoresis. *Ann. N. Y. Acad. Sci., 121*:350, 1964.

15. Polesky, H. F., Rokala, D., and Hoff, T.: "Serum Proteins in Paternity Testing," in *Paternity Testing.* Polesky, H. F. (ed.), Chicago, ASCP, 1975, p. 31-44.

16. Hirschfeld, J.: Immunoelectrophoretic demonstration of qualitative differences in normal human sera and their relation to the haptoglobins. *Acta Path. Microbiol. Scand., 47*:160, 1959.

17. Allison, A. C., and Blumberg, B. S.: An isoprecipitation reaction distinguishing human serum protein types. *Lancet,* i, 634, 1961.

18. Berg, K.: A new serum type system in man—the Lp system. *Acta Path. Microbiol. Scand., 59*:369, 1963.

19. Bradbrook, I. D., Grant, A., and Adinolfi, M.: Ag(x) and Ag(y) antigens in studies of paternity cases in the United Kingdom. *Human Heredity, 21*:493-499, 1971.

20. Fudenberg, H. H., Stiehm, E. R., Franklin, E. C., Meltzer, M., and Frangione, B.: Antigenicity of hereditary human gamma globulin (Gm) factors—biological and biochemical aspects. *Cold Spring Harbor Symposia on Quantitative Biology, 29*:463-472, 1964.

21. Schanfield, M. S., Polesky, H. F., and Sebring, E. S.: "Gm and Inv Typing," in *Paternity Testing*. Polesky, H. F. (ed.). Chicago, ASCP, 1975, p. 45-53.

22. Grubb, R.: *The Genetic Markers of Human Immunoglobulins*. New York, Springer-Verlag, 1970.

23. Ropartz, C.: L'allotypie des immunoglobulines humaines. *Ann. Immunol.*, *125*:27-39, 1974.

24. WHO Workshop. Rouen, France, 1974.

25. Schanfield, M. S., Gershowitz, H., and Ohkura, K.: Studies on the immunoglobulin allotypes of Asiatic populations. *Hum. Hered.*, *22*:496, 1972.

26. Schanfield, M. S., Gershowitz, H., Ohkura, K., and Blackwell, R. Q.: Studies on the immunoglobulin allotypes of Asiatic populations. *III Gm and Inv allotypes in Chinese*. *Hum. Hered.*, *22*:138, 1972.

27. Schanfield, M. S.: *Immunoglobulin haplotypes in Tlaxcalan and other populations in population studies on Tlaxcalans*. Crawford, M. (ed.) University of Kansas Press. In preparation, 1975.

28. Weitkamp, L. R., Salzant, F. M., Neel, J. V., Porta, F.; Geerdink, R. A., and Tarnoky, A. L.: Human serum albumin: twenty-three genetic variants and their population distribution. *Ann. Hum. Genet.*, Lond., *36*:381-392, 1973.

29. Dykes, D. D.: "Serum proteins and erythrocyte enzymes in paternity testing" in *AABB Technical Seminar*. R. Walker (Ed.), 1975.

30. Spencer, N., Hopkinson, D. A., and Harris, H.: Adenosine deaminase polymorphism in man. *Ann. Hum. Genet.*, *32*:9, 1968.

31. Wrede, B., Koops, E., and Brinkmann, B.: Determination of three enzyme polymorphisms in one electrophoretic step on horizontal polyacrylamide gels. *Humangenetik*, *13*:250, 1971.

32. Brinkmann, B., Brinkmann, M., and Martin, H.: A new allele in red cell adenosine deaminase polymorphism: ADA°. *Hum. Hered.*, *23*:603, 1973.

33. Chen, S-H., Scott, C. R., and Giblett, E. R.: Adenosine deaminase: demonstration of a "silent" gene associated with combined immunodeficiency disease. *Am. J. Hum. Genet.*, *26*:103-107, 1974.

34. Chen, S-H., Scott, C. R., and Swedberg, K. R.: Heterogeneity for adenosine deaminase deficiency: expression of the enzyme in cultured skin fibroblasts and amniotic fluid cells. *Am. J. Hum. Genet.*, *27*:46, 1975.

35. Dissing, J., and Knudsen, J. B.: A new red cell adenosine deaminase phenotype in man. *Hum. Hered.*, *19*:375, 1969.

36. Wüst, H.: The red cell adenosine deaminase (ADA) polymorphism in Vienna: distribution and usefulness in disputed parentage, preliminary report. *Vox Sang.*, *20*:267-270, 1971.

37. Chan, K. L.: Human red cell adenylate kinase polymorphism in West Malaysian populations. *Human Heredity, 21*:173-179, 1971.

38. Fildes, R. A., and Harris, H.: Genetically determined variation of adenylate kinase in man. *Nature, 209*:261-265, 1966.

39. Goedde, H. W., and Brenkmann, H-G.: GPT, 6-PGD, PGM and and AK phenotyping in one starch gel. *Humangenetik, 15*:277, 1972.

40. Rapley, S., Robson, E. B., Harris, H., and Smith, S. M.: Data on the incidence, segregation and linkage relation of the adenylate kinase (AK) polymorphism. *Ann. Hum. Genet., 31*:237, 1967.

41. Sørensen, S. A.: Adenylate kinase, adenosine deaminase and phosphoglucomutase phenotypes in a Danish population. *Human Heredity, 22*:362-371, 1972.

42. Brewer, G. J., and Dern, R. J.: A new inherited enzyme deficiency of human erythrocytes: 6-phosphogluconate dehydrogenase deficiency. *Am. J. Hum. Genet., 16*:472-476, 1964.

43. Fildes, R. A., and Parr, C. W.: Human red-cell phosphogluconate dehydrogenases. *Nature, 200*:890-891, 1963.

44. Blake, N. M., and Kirk, R. L.: New genetic variant of 6-phosphogluconate dehydrogenase in Australian Aborigines. *Nature, 221*:278, 1969.

45. Frischer, H., Bowman, J. E., Carson, P. E., Rieckmann, K. H., Willerson, D., and Colwell, E. J.: Erythrocyte glutathione reductase, glucose-6-phosphate dehydrogenase and 6-phosphogluconic dehydrogenase deficiencies in population of the United States, South Vietnam, Iran and Ethiopia. *J. Lab. Clin. Med., 81*:603-612, 1973.

46. Jenkins, T., and Nurse, G. T.: The red cell 6-phosphogluconate dehydrogenase polymorphism in certain Southern African populations; with the first report of a new phenotype. *Ann. Hum. Genet., 38*:19, 1974.

47. Luan Eng, L-I., and Welch, Q. B.: Electrophoretic variants of 6-phosphogluconate dehydrogenase (6-PGD) and phosphohexose isomerase (PHI) in different racial groups in Malaysia. *Human Heredity, 22*:338-343, 1972.

48. Tuchinda, S., Rucknagel, D. L., Na-Nakorn, S., and Wasi, P.: The Thai variant and the distribution of alleles of 6-phosphogluconate dehydrogenase and the distribution of glucose-6-phosphate dehydrogenase deficiency in Thailand. *Biochem. Genet., 2*:253, 1968.

49. Yunis, J. J.: *Biochemical Methods in Red Cell Genetics.* New York and London, Academic Press, 1969, pp. 354-368.

50. MacDonald, J. L.: Segregation analysis of three red cell isoenzymes. *Human Heredity, 21*:371-375, 1971.

51. Renninger, W., and Spielmann, W.: Beitrag zur genetik der erythrocy-tenphosphoglucomutase. *Humangenetik*, 8:64-66, 1969.

52. Brinkmann, B., Koops, E., Klopp, O., and Heindl, K.: Inherited partial deficiency of the $PGM_1{}^1$ gene: biochemical and densitometric studies. *Ann. Hum. Genet.*, London, 35:363-366, 1972.

53. Monn, E.: Application of the phosphoglucomutase (PGM) system of human red cells in paternity cases. *Vox Sang.*, 16:211-221, 1969.

54. Berg, K., Kamel, R., Schwarzfischer, F., and Wischerath, H.: The human red cell acid phosphatase activity and its statistical evaluation. *Humangenetik*, 24:213-215, 1974.

55. Fisher, R. A., and Harris H.: Studies on the separate isozymes of red cell acid phosphatase phenotypes A and B: II comparison of kinetics and stabilities of the isozymes. *Ann. Hem. Genet.*, London, 34:439-448, 1971.

56. Luffman, J. E., and Harris, H.: A comparison of some properties of human red cell acid phosphatase in different phenotypes. *Ann. Hum. Genet.*, 30:387-401, 1967.

57. Giblett, E. R., and Scott, N. M.: Red cell acid phosphatase: racial distribution and report of a new phenotype. *Am. J. Hum. Genet.*, 17:425-432, 1965.

58. Herbich, J., Fisher, R. A., and Hopkinson, D. A.: Atypical segregation of human red cell acid phosphatase phenotypes: evidence for a rare 'silent' allele P°. *Ann. Hum. Genet.*, 34:145, 1970.

59. Povey, S., and Swallow, D. M.: Probable assignment of the locus determining human red cell acid phosphatase ACP, to chromosome 2 using somatic cell hybrids. *Ann. Hum. Genet.*, London, 38:1-5, 1974.

60. Sørensen, S. A.: Report and characterization of a new variant EB, of human red cell acid phosphatase. *Am. J. Hum. Genet.*, 27:100, 1975.

61. Borman, P., Grundin, R., and Lins, P. E.: The red cell acid phosphatase polymorphism in Sweden: gene frequencies and application to disputed paternity. *Acta Genet. Med. Gemollol*, 20:77, 1971.

62. Fuhrmann, W. K., and Lichte, H.: Human red cell acid phosphastase polymorphism. A study of gene frequency and forensic use of the system in cases of disputed paternity. *Humangenetik*, 3:121, 1966.

63. Chen, S-H., and Giblett, E. R.: Polymorphism of soluble glutamic-pyruvic transaminase: a new genetic marker in man. *Science*, 173:148-149, 1971.

64. Kömpf, J., Bissbort, S., Ritter, H., and Wendt, G. G.: The polymorphism of alanine aminotransferase (E.C.2.6.1.2.): densitometric assay. *Humangenetik*, 22:247, 1974.

65. Olaisen, B.: Atypical segregation of erythrocyte glutamic-pyruvic

transaminase in a Norwegian family. *Hum. Hered., 23:*595-602, 1973.

66. Wiebecke, D., and Brackebusch, H. D.: Studies on the polymorphism of the soluble glutamic-pyruvic-transaminase in the population of Northern Bavaria (Germany). *Humangenetik, 23:*227-229, 1974.

67. Bender, K., and Frank, R.: Esterase D—Polymorphisms: Darstellung in der Hochspannungselektrophorese and Mitteilung von Allelhaufigkeiten. *Humangenetik, 23:*315-318, 1974.

68. Hopkinson, D. A., Mestriner, M. A., Cortner, J., and Harris, H.: Esterase D: a new human polymorphism. *Ann. Hum. Genet., 37:*119-137, 1973.

69. Ishimoto, G., Kuwata, M., and Fujita, H.: Esterase D polymorphism in Japanese. *Jap. J. Human Genet., 19:*157-160, 1974.

70. Welch, S.: Red cell esterase D polymorphism in Gambia. *Humangenetik, 21:*365, 1973.

71. Polesky, H. F., Dykes, D. D., Scarr-Salapatek, S., and Katz, S. H.: Unpublished observations.

72. Hirschfeld, J.: Immuno-electrophoretic demonstration of qualitative differences in human sera and their relation to the haptoglobins. *Acta Path. et Microbiol. Scand., 47:*160, 1959.

73. Kitchin, F. D.: Demonstration of the inherited serum group specific protein by acrylamide electrophoresis. *Proc. Soc. Exp. Biol. Med., 119:*1153, 1965.

74. Laurell, C. B.: Antigen-antibody crossed electrophoresis. *Ann. Biochem., 10:*358, 1965.

75. Sutcliffe, R. G., and Brock, D. J. H.: Group-specific component phenotyping by antibody-antigen crossed electrophoresis. *Biochem. Genet., 9:*63-68, 1973.

76. Cleve, H.: The variants of the group-specific component: a review of their distribution in human populations. *Israel J. Med. Sci., 9:*1133-1146, 1973.

77. Cleve, H., and Vavrusa, B.: Gc Opara: a variant of the group specific component (Gc) system with an electrophoretic mobility intermediate between Gc 1-1 and Gc 2-2. *Vox Sang., 26:*157-162, 1974.

78. Giblett, E. R.: *Genetic Markers in Human Blood.* London/Oxford, Blackwell, 1969.

79. Hirschfeld, J.; Honsson, B., and Rasmuson, M.: Inheritance of a new group-specific system demonstrated in normal human sera by means of an immuno-electrophoretic technique. *Nature, 185:*931, 1960.

80. Hirschfeld, J., and Heiken, A.: Application of the Gc system in paternity cases. *Am. J. Human Genet., 15:*19, 1963.

81. Reinskou, T.: Application of the Gc system in 1338 paternity cases. *Vox Sang., 11*:59, 1966.

82. McCombs, M. L., Bowman, B. H., and Alperin, J. B.: A new ceruloplasmin variant Cp Galveston. *Clin. Genet., 1*:30, 1970.

83. McCombs, M. L., and Bowman, B. H.: Demonstration of inherited ceruloplasmin variants in human serum by acrylamide electrophoresis. *Texas Reports on Biology and Medicine, 27*:769, 1969.

84. Shreffler, D. C., Brewer, G. J., Gall, J. C., and Honeyman, M. S.: Electrophoretic variation in human serum ceruloplasmin: a new genetic polymorphism. *Biochem. Genet., 1*:101, 1967.

85. McAlister, R., Martin, G. M., and Benditt, E. P.: Evidence for multiple ceruloplasmin variants in human serum. *Nature, 190*:927, 1961.

86. Roeser, H. P., Lee, G. R., Nacht, S. and Cartwright, G. E.: The role of ceruloplasmin in iron metabolism. *J. Clin. Invest., 49*:2408, 1970.

87. Shokier, M. H. K., and Shreffler, D. C.: "Characterization of ceruloplasmin variants: a proposed model for control of quantitative genetic expression." Abstract 12, Meet. Am. Soc. Hum. Genet., San Francisco, 1969.

88. Tanis, R. J., Neel, J. V., Dovey, H., and Morrow, M.: The genetic structure of a tribal population, the Yanomama Indians. IX. Gene frequencies for 18 serum proteins and erythrocyte systems in the Yanomama and five neighboring tribes: nine new variants. *Am. J. Hum. Genet., 25*:655, 1973.

89. Giblett, E. R., and Steinberg, A. G.: The inheritance of serum haptoglobin types in American Negroes: evidence for a third allele $Hp^{2m}$. *Amer. J. Hum. Genet., 12*:160-169, 1960.

90. Hauge, M., Heiken, A., and Höglund, C.: Studies on the haptoglobin system. II The development and distribution of Hp groups in children. *Human Heredity, 20*:557-565, 1970.

91. Sutton, H. E.: "The Haptoglobins" in *Progress in Medical Genetics*, Steinberg, A. G. and Bearn, A. G. (eds.). New York, Grune and Stratton, 1970, vol. 7, p. 163.

93. Beckman, L., Heiken, A., and Hirschfeld, J.: Frequency of haptoglobin types in the Swedish population. *Hereditas, 47*:599, 1961.

94. Poulik, M. D.: Starch gel electrophoresis in a discontinuous system of buffers. *Nature, 180*:1477, 1957.

95. Teisberg, P.: Transferrin variants in Norway. *Human Heredity, 22*:259-263, 1972.

96. Brönnestam, R.: Studies of C3 polymorphism: relationship between phenotype and quantitative immunochemical measurement. *Human Heredity, 23*:128-134, 1973.

97. Alper, C. A., Propp, R. P., Kemperer, M. R., and Rosen, F. S.: In-

herited deficiency of the third component of human complement (C'3). *J. Clin. Invest.*, *48*:553, 1969.

98. Brönnestam, R.: Studies of C3 polymorphism: distribution of C3 phenotypes in different areas of Sweden. *Human Heredity*, *23*:361-369, 1973.

99. Mauff, G., Freis, H., Potrafki, B. G., Hummel, K., and Pulverer, G.: Zur problematils der bestimmung seltener varianten des C3-polymorphism. *Humangenetik*, *22*:211-220, 1974.

100. Propp, R. P., and Alper, C. A.: C'3 Synthesis in human fetus and lack of transplacental passage. *Science*, *162*:672-673, 1968.

101. Teisberg, P.: New variants in the C3 system. *Hum. Hered.*, *20*:631-637, 1970.

102. Grubb, R.: Aggulination of erythrocytes coated with "incomplete" anti-Rh by certain rheumatoid arthritis sera and some other sera. The existence of human serum groups. *Acta Path. Microbiol. Scand.*, *39*:195, 1956.

103. Butler, R.: *Isoantigenicity of Human Plasma Proteins*. Bibliotheca Haematologica, No. 31. New York, S. Karger, 1969.

104. Natvig, J. B., and Kunkel, H. G.: Genetic markers of human immunoglobulins. The Gm and Inv systems. *Ser. Haematol.*, *1*:66, 1968.

105. Steinberg, A. G.: "Contribution of the Gm and Inv Allotypes to the Characterization of Human Populations," in *Genetic Polymorphisms and Diseases in Man*, Bracha Ramot (ed.). New York, Academic Press, 1974, pp. 123-130.

106. Ellis, F. R., Camp, F. R., and Litwin, S. D.: "Application of Gm typing to paternity exclusion." AABB 23rd annual meeting, San Francisco, 1970.

107. Harboe, M., and Lundevall, J.: The application of the Gm-system in paternity cases. *Vox Sang.*, *6*:257, 1961.

108. Pettenkofer, H. J., and Fiedler, H.: Eine versuchsandordnung zur sichesung von vaterschaftsausschlüssen im Gm- and Inv-system. *Blut*, *16*:225-226, 1968.

109. Rokala, D. A.: "The anthropological genetics and demography of the Southwestern Ojibwa in the Greater Leech Lake-Chippewa National Forest area." PhD thesis, Univ. of Minn., 1971.

# CHAPTER SEVEN

# LIKELIHOOD OF PARENTAGE

ALEXANDER S. WIENER

I<small>N</small> U<small>NITED</small> S<small>TATES</small> <small>COURTS</small> blood grouping tests are ordinarily used as exclusionary evidence of parentage only. For example, when the mother is group O and her baby is group A, if the man accused of paternity is group B this is accepted by courts as conclusive proof that the accused man is not the father of the child in question, and the defendant is exonerated. On the other hand, in a similar case in which the mother is group O and her child A, if the defendant is group A or group AB so that paternity is not excluded, the findings are considered inconclusive since almost 50 percent of all men are group A or AB, and the results are therefore not admissible in evidence.

Suppose, however, that the mother is group O and her child is subgroup $A_3$ and the accused man is also subgroup $A_3$. Such a finding, which does not exclude paternity, can hardly be dismissed without further notice in the interest of justice. Subgroup $A_3$ is so rare that its coincidental presence in a child and a man accused of his paternity should be considered strong circumstantial evidence that the defendant actually is the father of the child. While such a case has never been reported, there have been comparable cases where the mother was type M and her child type $MN_2$ and the defendant also type $MN_2$, especially in Chinese among whom the rare type $MN_2$ has a higher frequency than among Whites or Blacks. Similarly, there have been cases in which the mother was type rh, her child type $Rh_z$rh and the accused man type $Rh_zRh_1$. In all such cases, i.e. where the accused and the baby both have rare genes such as $N^2$ or $R^z$ (or $r^y$), absent in the mother, it has been the custom to call the facts to the attention of the court and to point out that the findings constituted strong circumstantial evidence, though not absolute proof, that the defendant actually was the father of the child.

In recent years, there has been an explosion in the knowledge of the blood and serum groups, haptoglobin types and isozymes, which have a clear-cut heredity and therefore yield findings theoretically applicable to problems of disputed parentage. In European countries, many of these newer tests are already being applied routinely, and many European courts are no longer satisfied with the use of blood tests only for exclusion; where the defendant in a paternity action is not excluded, they expect the expert to render a report as to the likelihood that the accused man actually is the father. The authors propose here to explain how blood tests are being applied for calculations of likelihood of paternity (as well as for exclusion of paternity) and to point out the limitations even when properly applied.

To compute the likelihood of paternity, $W$, one must take into account the *a priori* probability of paternity, $P_A$, and the chance, $P_E$, that a man falsely accused of paternity would be excluded by at least one of the tests used. The value of $P_A$, depends on the experience of the courts—e.g., if 75 percent of the defendants have been found to be innocent of the charge, then the *a priori* probability of paternity, $P_A$, is 0.75. Moreover, if n independent tests are carried out which have the respective chances, $P_1$, $P_2$, $P_3$, and $P_n$, of excluding paternity of a falsely accused man, then

$$P_E = 1 - (1 - P_1)(1 - P_2)(1 - P_3) \ldots (1 - P_n)$$

It is easy to show the likelihood of paternity, $W$, is given by the formula

$$W = \frac{P_A}{P_A + (1 - P_A)(1 - P_E)}$$

When the *a priori* probability of paternity, $P_A$, is one half (50%), this formula reduces to

$$W = \frac{1}{2 - P_E}$$

Two cases will be described which illustrate the usefulness and limitations of such calculations of likelihood of paternity.

## Case 1

In this case, the mother stated she had had sexual relations with two (and only two) men and was herself uncertain which of the two men was the father of her child. Here, therefore, it may be assumed that the *a priori* probability of paternity was 0.5 for both of the accused men. Blood grouping tests yielded the following results:

| Blood of | A-B-O Groups | M-N Type | Kell Type | Rh-Hr Type |
|---|---|---|---|---|
| Mother ..................... | B | MN | k | $Rh_1rh$ |
| Child ...................... | $A_2$ | MN | k | $Rh_1rh$ |
| 1st man ..................... | $A_1$ | MN | k | $Rh_zRh_o$ |
| 2nd man ..................... | $A_2$ | MN | k | $Rh_1rh$ |

As can be seen, neither of the two men was excluded by the blood grouping tests. The court, of course, was interested in knowing whether the results threw any light at all on the problem, and for this the tests for the subgroups of group A appeared especially worthy of notice.

Since the mother was group B and her child was subgroup $A_2$, the child was a carrier of gene $A^2$, which had to be derived from his father. The group $A_1$ defendant could belong to any of the three genotypes $A^1A^1$, $A^1A^2$ or $A^1O$, while the group $A_2$ defendant had to belong to either genotype $A^2A^2$ or genotype $A^2O$. Taking the gene frequencies for the general population to be $O = 0.672$, $A^1 = 0.179$, $A^2 = 0.057$ and $B = 0.091$, the chances that the group $A_1$ defendant would produce a sperm cell carrying gene $A^2 = \frac{1}{2}A^1A^2/(A^1A^1 + A^1A^2 + A^1O) = 0.0102/(0.0320 + 0.2409 + 0.0204) = 0.03475$. Similarly, the chance that the group $A_2$ defendant would produce an $A^2$ sperm cell $= (\frac{1}{2}A^2O + A^2A^2)/A^2O + A^2A^2) = (0.0383 + 0.003251)/(0.0767 + 0.00325) = 0.5203$. Thus, the odds that it was the group $A_2$ man rather than the $A_1$ man who fathered the child was 0.5203 to 0.03425 or about 15 to 1. This information was transmitted to the court, but the final disposal of the case is not known to the authors.

In conclusion, it should be mentioned that while the two men belonged to the same M-N and Kell type, their Rh-Hr types differed. The child who was type $Rh_1rh$ could have obtained either his $R^1$ (or $r'$) or his $r$ (or $R^o$) gene from his mother who was also type $Rh_1rh$. If the latter, his $R^1$ (or $r'$) gene would have had to come from his father, and both accused men could provide that gene with equal likelihood. If, on the other hand, the child had obtained his $R^1$ (or $r'$) gene from his mother then his $r$ (or $R^o$) gene would have to have been derived from the father. In that case, the first man was excluded as the possible father except in the unlikely event that he was subtype $Rh_zrh$ instead of the usual subtype $Rh_1Rh_2$. These considerations increase further the likelihood that the second man was the father of the child rather than the first man.

## Case 2

In this second case, there also were two and only two men either one of whom, the mother stated, could be the father of her child. However, only one of the two men was available for testing, and the results of the tests on the mother, child, and the man in question were as follows:

| Blood of | A-B-O Group | M-N Type | Kell Type | Rh-Hr Type |
|---|---|---|---|---|
| Mother | O | M | k | $Rh_1Rh_2$ |
| Child | $A_1$ | MN | K | $Rh_1Rh_1$ |
| Putative father | $A_1$ | MN | K | $Rh_1Rh_1$ |

Obviously, the findings did not exclude paternity; instead as can readily be shown, they strongly indicated that the man tested was indeed the father of the child. It is noteworthy, that the child had the agglutinogens $A_1$, N, and K which were lacking from the mother's blood, so that the child's father had to have all three factors $A_1$, N, and K. In addition, since the child was type $Rh_1Rh_1$ his father had to have the factor rh'. The chance that a man selected at random from the general population would have all four factors, $A_1$, N, K, and rh' is the product of their frequencies, i.e. $(0.33)(0.70)(0.084)(0.70) = 0.01358$. In other words, the chance that a falsely accused man would lack at least one of the four factors and therefore be excluded was $P_E = 1 - 0.01358 = 0.9864$. Since there were two possible fathers, the *a priori* probability of paternity $P_A = 0.5$. Therefore, the likelihood of paternity, $W = \frac{1}{2 - 0.9864}$, or about 74 to 1, approximately. The court was so informed.

Nothing further was heard of the case until two-and-a-half years later, when the court sent the second man for testing. This man proved to be group $A_1$, type MN, type K, and type $Rh_1rh$, so that the second man was not excluded either, contrary to expectations. Thus, in the final report to the court, the authors had to point out that likelihood of paternity was almost the same for the two men, and that the completed findings were inconclusive as to the problem of paternity. This case, therefore, illustrates the danger of conclusions based on calculations of likelihood of paternity, and the court must be constantly alert to these limitations if miscarriage of justice is to be averted.

## LIMITATIONS OF ATTEMPTS TO DETERMINE THE LIKELIHOOD OF PATERNITY

Theoretically, the application in combination of multiple tests, each of which has the potential to exclude parentage, as evidence of the likelihood of paternity has the limitation that the ideal of excluding 100 percent of falsely accused men can theoretically never be attained, though this objective can be approximated as closely as desired provided that there are enough reliable tests all of which can be done. Suppose that by doing a set of a score of separate tests, 99 percent of falsely accused men can be exonerated, while by using another set of a score of different tests, 99 percent of innocent men can also be exonerated. Then, by doing all forty tests in combination, there will still be some few falsely accused men who will not be excluded by any of the tests. It is clear that the chance that a falsely accused man will not be excluded by any of the first set of twenty tests is .01 or 1 percent, while the chance of nonexclusion by the second set of tests is also .01, so that even if all forty tests are done the chance of excluding paternity is 99.99 percent and not 100 percent because .01 × .01 = .0001 or one hundredth of one percent of falsely accused men would not be excluded by any of the forty tests used.

Obviously, attempts to push the number of tests done to the point where even only 99 percent (if not all) falsely accused men will be excluded by the tests is both impractical and impracticable. Suppose that enough tests have been done to exclude 90 percent of falsely accused men and it is proposed to do still another test offering a 10 percent exclusion rate. Since of the men excluded by such an additional test 90 percent will already have been excluded by at least one of the other tests, the new test would raise the exclusion rate only from 90 to 91 percent. Thus, at this level, the accused man derives only one tenth of the potential value of any new test, for the same cost. Consequently, not only is it impracticable to push the number of tests done in order to achieve the ideal of 99 percent exclusions, but the high cost would render this impractical. Obviously, no fixed level can be set for routine use, and the number of tests done will depend on the circumstances. For practical purposes, one may have to be content to achieve an exclusion rate of 90 percent or even much lower, though in cases involving wealthy individuals, for example, in an inheritance case of a millionaire, it may be desirable to use every available test which can throw light on the problem of parentage. In this country, for routine court cases of disputed paternity, it has been the general practice for practical purposes to limit the tests to the six A-B-O blood groups and subgroups, the three M-N types, and the Rh-Hr system, which in combination will exclude no more than 55 percent of falsely accused men.

Another and more serious limitation of attempts to determine likelihood of paternity by multiple tests is the danger of errors and resulting miscarriage of justice. Even at the time when the only tests available were with anti-**A** and anti-**B** sera, so that blood tests for forensic problems of paternity were limited to the four A-B-O blood groups, there was evidence that mistakes in blood grouping were plentiful so that there must have been cases in which miscarriage of justice resulted where the tests were in error and falsely excluded an accused man.[1] Even in recent years, despite the ready commercial availability of antisera of high potency and specificity, such errors continue to occur. In one such case the mother was reported to be group O, the child group A and the accused man group B and paternity was said to be excluded; actually the defendant was group AB, subgroup $A_2B$ and the child was subgroup $A_2$ which was circumstantial evidence that the man really was the father. Similarly, in a kidnapping case, the woman accused of the crime was reported to be group B and the baby group O; actually the kidnapper proved to be subgroup A$_2$B which proved that she was not the mother of the baby which she claimed was her own.

Obviously, if errors and miscarriages of justice are to be avoided, only fully qualified individuals should be permitted to carry out the tests and testify as to the results. Unfortunately, this ideal does not prevail and researchers have had occasion to retest and have detected errors in more than a score of cases in which the petitioner (mother of the baby) protested when the report of the first "expert" excluded paternity falsely.[2] In these cases, the errors had to do with the M-N typing or Rh Hr typing of the blood specimens. If the newer tests are included, the possibility of error will, of course, be multiplied, especially because many of the newer tests are not fully perfected. It must be borne in mind that there are few if any individuals and laboratories who are qualified and technically equipped and prepared to carry out all the tests which have been described in the literature. The number of errors which occur can be kept at a minimum only if every expert consulted by the courts limits his report to those tests for which that expert is fully qualified by study and experience. Unfortunately, there are experts who seem unable to resist the temptation to carry out tests not yet fully perfected and which they are not fully qualified to do, in order to make their report as "complete" as possible. To be sure, the more tests that are done the greater the chances of excluding paternity, but as the number of tests increase the chances of exclusion of paternity increase more and more slowly, while the costs inexorably increase as does the likelihood of error. Finally, a point will be reached at which the chances of exclusion increase more slowly even than the chances of error and where further testing is extravagantly costly and is insufficiently rewarding.

Fortunately, with the availability of air mail, free resort to the use of consultation is possible. Every expert should limit his tests to those in which he is fully qualified, and in cases where further testing is desired, he should mail the blood specimens to other experts and consultation laboratories properly qualified to carry out those tests. Also, every exclusion or calculation of probability of paternity should preferably be checked by at least one other independent qualified expert. Only if such precautions are adhered to will the full potential of modern tests for parentage and nonparentage be realized, without the danger of errors and miscarriage of justice.

### REFERENCES

1. Wiener, A. S.: Forensic blood group genetics. *N. Y. State J. Med.*, 72:810-815, 1972.
2. Wiener, A. S.: Problems and pitfalls in blood grouping tests for disputed parentage. II. The Rh-Hr blood group system. *J. Forensic Med.* (S. Afr.), 15:106-132, 1968.

# CHAPTER EIGHT

# MEDICOLEGAL USES FOR BLOOD GROUPING TESTS

LEON N. SUSSMAN

## PRINCIPLES

THE RELIABILITY of the transmission of the genes that determine the blood groups and the immutability of these blood groups have motivated their use in solving many problems in forensic medicine. No other human characteristics are so secure from environmental influences as are the blood groups, for they cannot be affected by age, diet, climate, radiation, or other common influences. Rare exceptions have been reported where a group A person has developed a transient weak **B** antigen on the red cells, while retaining unchanged their usual anti-**B** agglutinin. These few exceptions were patients severely ill with diseases such as acute leukemia, widespread carcinomatosis, or virulent bacteremias. Replacement transfusion, performed principally in erythroblastosis fetalis, can produce a temporary change in the blood groups; however, within a few weeks the foreign transfused blood is again replaced by the patient's own blood with the patient's original blood type.

Blood tests are of value in a negative way—they may indicate that a man is *not* the father of a child, or that a relationship does *not* exist. Attempts to prove such a relationship cannot be positive, although the presence of a rare gene in a child and in his alleged father would indicate a high probability of parentage. Thus, the rare gene $M^g$ (frequency 1:40,000) or $r^y$ (frequency 1:10,000) or $r^{wi}$ (frequency 1:20,000), if found in both child and putative father, would strongly suggest paternity. The possibility of coincidence being responsible is so remote as to make the odds astronomical. Such a presumption of paternity can be used as

132

strong supportive evidence but not as the basis for a definite conclusion.

In some cases the overwhelming likelihood of paternity by combinations of unusual blood types is convincing although never absolute. Chapter Seven deals with the methods and value of such probabilities and the necessary precautions and risks that are involved.

A courtroom rebuttal frequently offered is that of the possibility that a mutation might have been the cause of the contradiction to the laws of theoretical expectancy. It is known that the mutation rate in humans is extremely small—in the nature of 1 in 50,000 gene generations[1] and that multiple somatic effects are usually present if the mutation has not been lethal. Only one such case has been reported in blood group studies, and that child had many congenital defects.[2] This certainly should prove the incredibility of such a line of argument.

## AREAS OF APPLICATION

There are many areas where blood grouping tests are of use in solving medicolegal problems. These include:

1. personal identification
2. differentiation between identical and fraternal twins
3. filial relationships
   a) mixed babies
   b) kidnapped children
   c) parentage studies
      1) parenthood claimed
      2) disputed paternity
      3) undisputed paternity
      4) maternal exclusions
4. identification of blood stains and body secretions
5. anthropology, population drifts.

### Personal Identification

The numerous possible combinations of the blood factors of each blood group system result in a number of blood types that almost insures the individuality of every person's blood. This is

TABLE 8-I

INDIVIDUALITY ATTAINABLE BY BLOOD GROUPING TESTS

| Systems | Phenotypes | Cumulative Totals |
|---|---|---|
| A-B-O | 6 | 6 |
| M-N-S-s | 9 | 54 |
| P | 3 | 162 |
| Rh-Hr | 28 | 4,536 |
| Kell | 5 | 25,000* |
| Duffy | 4 | 100,000 |
| Lewis | 4 | 400,000 |
| Kidd | 3 | 1,200,000 |
| Lutheran | 3 | 3,600,000 |
| Diego | 2 | 7,200,000 |
| Vel | 2 | 14,400,000 |
| Yt$^a$ | 2 | 28,800,000 |
| Xg$^a$ | 2 | 57,600,000 |

* From Kell to Xg$^a$ cumulative totals are approximated.

true, except for identical twins, since coming from the same fertilized ovum they must inherit the identical genes. By the use of the available serums, it is possible to construct Table 8-I which indicates cumulatively the number of individual blood types that can be differentiated.[3]

The table must now be further expanded by the use of plasma proteins and erythrocyte isoenzymes with demonstrable characteristics as described in Chapter Six.

Another aspect of identification by means of blood grouping tests is based on the discovery that certain blood types are limited to separate racial groups. Thus, the factors **hr**$^V$, **Js**$^a$, and the blood type Fy$^{(a-b-)}$ are found almost exclusively in Negroes; the factor **Di**$^a$ found only in South American Indians, Japanese, and Chinese; and the factor **Xg**$^a$ found only on the X chromosome.

### Fraternal and Identical Twins

This differentiation between twin pairs is no problem if they are of opposite sex. When the twins are of the same sex, their proper classification may require detailed blood group analysis. Monozygotic twins, coming from a single ovum, must have identical blood group factors for every system being tested. Any single difference indicates nonidentity. The mathematical probability of solving this problem has been calculated by several geneticists;[4, 5, 6, 7] and depends, of course, upon the number of blood groups that are tested and their distribution.

## Filial Relationship

The most frequent medicolegal use of blood grouping tests is in some aspect of filial relationship, usually involving the paternity of a child. Many states have statutes that make the results of such tests "decisive of the issue" if paternity is excluded. In other states, if an exclusion is found, the results are considered "most reliable evidence." A uniform act on blood tests to determine paternity has been proposed.* The legal aspects of such proceedings are thoroughly detailed in the book, *Disputed Paternity Proceedings*[8] by S. B. Schatkin, former Assistant Corporation Counsel of the City of New York.

The Committee on Medicolegal Problems of the American Medical Association[9] has recommended the use of only the A-B-O, M-N, and Rh-Hr systems in parentage proceedings. The result of the tests in the other blood group systems may be admissible as evidence when performed by those who have the necessary experience with the special reagents that are needed. The committee has also outlined the qualifications of such experts in the field of immunohematology and has prepared lists of such experts which are available from the Law Department of the A.M.A. It must be emphasized that these delicate tests and their proper interpretation regarding paternity are not the province of the ordinary clinical laboratory. Results submitted as legal evidence must be supported by an expert who can withstand the necessary cross-examination regarding his skill, experience, knowledge, and technics in order to warrant valid consideration. The laboratories of such experts are easily available by air transportation, when corroboration of such findings is advisable.

---

* A Uniform Act on Blood Tests to Determine Paternity by the National Conference of the Commission on Uniform State Laws was approved in San Francisco in 1952, and it is now incorporated into the statutes of many states.

## Mixed Babies

The problem deals with the rare complaint that newborn babies may have been interchanged in the hospital nursery. This highly charged emotional situation can usually be quickly resolved by blood grouping tests of the two infants and the two sets of parents. With the combined use of the A-B-O, M-N, and Rh-Hr tests, the chance of correctly sorting out the families is over 90 percent. Wiener has reported such a situation[10] in which the first set of parents were both of group O, and the second set were group O (father) and group AB (mother). Since one of the infants was group A, this baby could only have been the child of the second set of parents. The other child, being of group O, therefore belonged to the first set of parents.

## Kidnapped Children

In these cases, the kidnapper usually claims she is the mother of the child who was born without benefit of professional help and, therefore, does not possess a birth certificate. Frequently, a "friend" is produced as the father. Since the blood of all the persons involved including the child, the kidnapper, the friend, and the parents can be tested, the results usually demonstrate quite clearly the falsity of the explanation. Two such cases have been reported[10] and are reproduced with the permission of the author.

The results of the blood tests were clear.

| CASE 1: | Father | A | MN | $Rh_1Rh_1$ |
|---------|--------|---|-----|-----------|
| | Mother | A | MN | $Rh_1Rh_1$ |
| | Baby | A | N | $Rh_1Rh_1$ |
| | Kidnapper Suspect | B | MN | $Rh_2Rh_2$ |
| | Friend of kidnapper suspect | O | MN | $Rh_1Rh_1$ |

The suspected kidnapper who claimed that she was the mother of the baby, and her friend whom she claimed to be the father, could not be the parents of the child. There was a double exclusion of maternity in that a $Rh_2Rh_2$ mother must transmit one of these factors to her child, and an $Rh_1Rh_1$ child must have obtained one of these factors from each of its parents. In addition, a mother of Group B and a father of Group O could not produce a child of Group A. On the other hand, there existed no evidence of exclusion between the true parents and the baby.

| CASE 2: | Father | O | MN | rh"rh |
|---------|--------|---|-----|-------|
| | Mother | O | MN | $Rh_1$rh |
| | Infant | O | M | $Rh_1$rh |
| | Suspect | $A_2$B | MN | $Rh_1Rh_2$ |

In this case, the A-B-O system excluded the kidnapper as the mother of the child, since an AB parent cannot have an O child.

## Parentage Studies

PARENTHOOD CLAIMED (ESTATE AND IMMIGRATION PROBLEMS): The situation where parentage is an issue has several ramifications. Occasionally, a claim is made that an unrecognized child (usually illegitimate) was deprived of his lawful inheritance. Such claims may be resolved by comparing the results of the blood grouping tests of the claimant and the deceased. If the tests of the second parent are also available, the possibility of excluding a false claim is greatly increased.

In another dramatic situation, an extremely high number of visa applications from Chinese males, who claimed Chinese-American citizens as their parents, led to the study of the blood groups of the "families." The high rate of exclusions that was obtained alerted the Immigration and Naturalization Service to the activities of an "immigration ring."[11, 12] Several examples of exclusions obtained in the study of Chinese applicants are listed in Table 8-II.

DISPUTED PATERNITY: The greatest number of blood grouping tests involves the question of disputed paternity. The usual problem relates to out-of-wedlock children where the man, alleged to be the father, denies the charge. A similar situation may be found in divorce proceedings where the husband charges his wife with adultery and denies the paternity of the children. A less common case exists in criminal rape proceedings where pregnancy results—the finding of an exclusion of paternity could absolve the suspect.

TABLE 8-II

PARENTAGE EXCLUSION (CHINESE IMMIGRATION CASES)
STUDY OF CHINESE APPLICANTS

| | Putative Father | Mother | | Applicant | Interpretation |
|---|---|---|---|---|---|
| Case I | O M Rh$_1$Rh$_1$ | A$_1$N Rh$_1$rh | | O MN Rh$_1$Rh$_2$ | Paternity Excluded (rh″) |
| Case II | A$_1$M Rh$_1$Rh$_1$ | Not available | (1) | A$_1$N Rh$_1$Rh$_1$ | Paternity Excluded (M-N) |
| | | | (2) | A$_1$M Rh$_1$Rh$_1$ | Paternity Not Excluded |
| Case III | A$_1$MN Rh$_1$Rh$_1$ | A$_1$B MN Rh$_2$Rh$_0$ | (1) | A$_1$N Rh$_1$Rh$_1$ | Paternity Not Excluded |
| | | | (2) | O Rh$_1$Rh$_2$ | Maternity Excluded (A-B-O) |
| Case IV | O N Rh$_1$Rh$_1$ | Not available | (1) | O M Rh$_1$rh | Paternity Excluded (M-N) |
| | | | (2) | O N Rh$_1$rh | Paternity Not Excluded |
| Case V | O N Rh$_2$rh | Not available | (3) | O MN Rh$_1$Rh$_1$ | Paternity Excluded (rh′-hr′) |

The area of disputed paternity has provided the largest body of statistics in the medicolegal application of blood grouping tests. In America, papers on this subject have been published by Wiener,[13, 18] Alvarez,[14] Unger,[15] Sussman,[16, 17, 19] and Marsters.[20] European experiences have been reported by Andresen,[21] Orth and Hirth,[22] Barandun et al.,[23] and Henningsen.[24] In New York City, the reports reveal that 16 percent of the defendants who deny the charge of paternity can be excluded as the father by blood tests. The chance that the combined tests A-B-O, M-N-S, and Rh-Hr will exclude a falsely accused man is approximately 53 percent[25] (with the additional test now available, 67% [Table 1-I]). Therefore, if sixteen out of 100 defendants can be excluded by these tests that are only 53 percent efficient, then approximately thirty-five out of 100 of the men in this series must have been falsely accused. An additional significant statistic is the finding that about 10 percent of the women making the charge failed to appear for the blood test when so ordered by the court—a situation which must be considered suspect.[19] Table 8-III records the results obtained in one of the series involving 1,000 cases[26] which yielded approximately the same percentage of results.

Thus, blood grouping tests in disputed paternity proceedings are capable of resolving the question in a significant percentage of cases where a man is falsely accused. Every defendant, therefore, should be offered the opportunity to benefit from such conclusive evidence.

UNDISPUTED PATERNITY (PATERNITY ADMITTED): Another aspect of the value of blood grouping tests in paternity proceedings was

TABLE 8-III

EXCLUSION OF PATERNITY

|  | No. of Cases | Percentage |
|---|---|---|
| Total completed cases | 1,000 | |
| Exclusion of paternity | 145 | 14.5 |
| Prob. of exclusion (A-B-O, M-N, Rh-Hr) | | 53 |
| Total probable exclusion | 284 | 28.4 |
| Total "no show"* | 112 | 11.2 |
| Total no. of men probably falsely accused | 396 | 39.6 |

* Women failed to appear.

disclosed in a paper by Sussman and Schatkin.[27] The tests were performed on the litigants after paternity was admitted and the cases legally closed. In this series, 9 percent of the men were shown by blood tests not to be the fathers of the children for whom they admitted paternity. Since the efficiency of these tests using only the standard A-B-O, M-N, and Rh-Hr system is approximately 50 percent, therefore, about 18 percent of all men admitting paternity in the New York City courts are really not the fathers of the children they accept as theirs.

In the interests of justice and truth, it has been recommended that blood tests be made mandatory as a prerequisite to the commencement of paternity proceedings.[28] In this way, the exposure to notoriety, defamation of character, and even blackmail—not to mention the high costs of legal defense—would be avoided for those wrongfully accused men who make up a considerable portion of the defendants in these actions.

MATERNAL EXCLUSIONS: The determination of nonpaternity assumes that the woman in the proceedings is truly the child's mother. The expression, "maternity is a fact whereas paternity is only an opinion," has been the basis for this assumption. On rare occasions, however, the blood grouping tests have excluded the mother. Case III (Table 8-II) presents such an example in which a child of Group O is claimed by a Group AB mother. Other similar situations were presented by Wiener.[10] The exclusion of maternity is an occasional finding in immigration cases where families were separated for years and substitution of children, either deliberate or accidental, took place. In the confusion of mass population movements such as war refugees and displaced groups, accidental interchange of babies is not inconceivable. Blood grouping tests can be useful in dispelling doubts by at least indicating that an exclusion does not exist, even though a filial relationship cannot be proven.

EXAMPLES OF EXCLUSION:

Exclusions of Paternity

A-B-O Exclusions:

| Case No. 2764: | Alleged Father | $A_1B$ | M | $Rh_1rh$ | K neg. | S neg. |
|---|---|---|---|---|---|---|
| | Mother | O | M | $Rh_1rh$ | K pos. | S pos. |
| | Child | O | M | $Rh_0$ | K neg. | S pos. |

An AB father must transmit the gene for either the A or B agglutinogen to his child. Since the alleged father is Group AB and the child is Group O possessing neither **A** nor **B**, paternity is excluded.

Case No. 2582:

| | | | | |
|---|---|---|---|---|
| Alleged Father | O | MN | $Rh_1rh$ | K neg. |
| Mother | O | M | $Rh_1rh$ | K neg. |
| Child | B | MN | $Rh_o$ | K neg. |

A child cannot have a blood factor not present in either his mother or father. Since the child is Group B, and the mother and the alleged father are Group O (lacking the **B** factor) paternity is excluded.

Rh-Hr Exclusions:

Case No. 2537:

| | | | | |
|---|---|---|---|---|
| Alleged Father | B | MN | $Rh_1Rh_1$ | K neg. |
| Mother | O | N | $Rh_o$ | K neg. |
| Child | O | MN | rh | K neg. |

An **hr′**-negative father (type $Rh_1Rh_1$) cannot have an **rh′**-negative (type rh) child. Paternity, therefore, is excluded.

Explanation: It is necessary, however, to prove that $\overline{\overline{Rh}}_o$ (double bar **Rh**$_o$) is not present, since the reactions would be similar if the father's genotype was $R^1\overline{\overline{R}}$. To avoid a false conclusion, the following test for $\overline{\overline{Rh}}_o$ should be performed:
1. The alleged father's and the child's red blood cells are tested in *saline* with incomplete (conglutinating) anti-**Rh**$_o$ serum. The reaction would be negative with cells having the normal **Rh**$_o$ factor, but would be positive if $\overline{\overline{Rh}}_o$ was present.
2. The child's cells are tested with serial dilutions of a saline anti-**hr′** serum to determine the presence of a single or double dose of the **hr′** factor (dosage effect). If a double dose of **hr′** is present, the exclusion of paternity is corroborated. This test is controlled by known cells, homozygous and heterozygous for **hr′**.

Titration Results:                              **hr′** Titer   Score   Interpretation

| | | hr′ Titer | Score | Interpretation |
|---|---|---|---|---|
| | Child's cells | 64 | 17 | 2 doses |
| | Father's cells | 0 | 0 | 0 |
| | Mother's cells | 64 | 17 | 2 doses |
| | Control cells | 4 | 6 | 1 dose |

Conclusion: $\overline{\overline{Rh}}_o$ (double bar **Rh**$_o$) is not present. The child has 2 doses of **hr′** whereas the putative father has none. The exclusion of paternity, therefore, is corroborated.

| Case No. 2719: | Alleged Father | O | N rh | K neg. S neg. |
|---|---|---|---|---|
| | Mother | A$_1$ | MN Rh$_2$rh | K neg. S neg. |
| | Child | A$_1$ | MN Rh$_1$rh | K neg. S neg. |

The blood factor **rh′** cannot be present in the blood of a child unless it is present in the blood of one or both parents. Since the child is **rh′**-positive and the alleged father and the mother are **rh′**-negative, paternity is excluded.

| Case No. 2613: | Alleged Father | B | M | Rh$_o$ | K neg. |
|---|---|---|---|---|---|
| | Mother | O | MN | Rh$_1$rh | K neg. |
| | Child | O | MN | Rh$_1$Rh$_1$ | K neg. |

A child of type Rh$_1$Rh$_1$ (homozygous for **rh′**) cannot have a parent who is **rh′**-negative. Since the alleged father is **rh′**-negative, paternity is excluded. Corroboration is necessary by proving the absence of **Rh**$_o$ (double bar **Rh**$_o$) and demonstrating the presence of a double dose of **rh′** in the child's blood by titration and scoring.

| Case No. 2449: | Alleged Father | B MN Rh$_z$Rh$_o$ | K neg. **hr** neg. |
|---|---|---|---|
| | Mother | A M  Rh$_z$Rh$_o$ | K neg. **hr** neg. |
| | Child | B MN Rh$_1$rh | K neg. **hr** pos. |

Both parents were **hr**$^-$-negative. Paternity, therefore, was excluded.

| Explanation: | The phenotype Rh$_z$Rh$_o$ indicates several possible genotypes—the most frequent being $R^1R^2$. The possibility of the genotype $R^zr$ also exists, in |
|---|---|

which case a child of phenotype $Rh_1rh$ could result. This can be tested by the use of anti-**hr** serum, which reacts with the gene products of $R^o$ and $r$. Thus if $R^zr$ was the true genotype of either parent, there would be agglutination (positive reaction) with anti-**hr**. Since the tests were negative, paternity is excluded.

Case No. 2644:

| | | | |
|---|---|---|---|
| Alleged Father | $A_1$ | N | $Rh_o$ |
| Mother | $A_1$ | N | $Rh_2Rh_2$ |
| Child | $A_1$ | N | rh |

In this case the alleged mother is **hr″**-negative, indicating that she is homozygous for the **rh″** factor. The child lacks **rh″**. Titration and scoring tests indicated that the mother possessed 2 **rh″** factors, whereas the child had none. An exclusion of maternity is, therefore, present. Maternal exclusions are quite rare but have been found in blood tests performed in proceedings involving derivative citizenship and disputed maternity in child kidnapping cases.

*M-N Exclusion*

Case No. 2673:

| | | | | |
|---|---|---|---|---|
| Alleged Father | $A_1$ | M | rh | K neg. |
| Mother | $A_1$ | M | $Rh_1rh$ | K neg. |
| Child | $A_1$ | MN | $Rh_1rh$ | K neg. |

A child who is group M-N must have inherited an *M* gene from one parent and an *N* gene from the other parent. Since the alleged father and the mother are type M (lacking *N*), paternity is excluded.

Case No. 2840:

| | | | | | |
|---|---|---|---|---|---|
| Alleged Father | $A_1$ | Nss | $M^g$ pos. | $Rh_2rh$ | K neg. |
| Mother | $A_1$ | MSs | $M^g$ neg. | $Rh_2rh$ | K neg. |
| Child | $A_1$ | MSs | $M^g$ pos. | $Rh_2rh$ | K neg. |

This is a very rare case that appears to be an M-N exclusion; however the presence of $M^g$ factor in both alleged father and child practically proves paternity.

Case No. 2768:  Alleged Father A₁  M      $Rh_zRh_o$  K neg  S neg.
                Mother          A   MN     $Rh_o$      K neg. S neg.
                Child           O   N      $Rh_1rh$    K neg. S neg.

A father of group M cannot have a child of group N. Paternity is, therefore, excluded. In this type of exclusion, if practicable, tests should be done for the factor $M^g$, since in very rare cases the alleged father's genotype could be $MM^g$ and the child's genotype $NM^g$. Although extremely rare (frequently estimated as 1:40,000), testing with anti-$M^g$ serum would eliminate this very small possibility. (*Cf.* Case No. 2840) Titrations to determine single or double doses of either M or N can be done in absence of anti-$M^g$ serum.

Case No. 2843:  Alleged Father A₁  MN  rh       K neg. S neg.
                Mother          A₁  M   $Rh_1rh$  K neg. S neg.
                Child           O   M   $Rh_1rh$  K neg. S pos.

A child who is S-positive must have inherited the gene for the S agglutinogen from either of his parents. Since both the alleged father and the mother are S-negative, paternity is excluded.

*Kell Exclusions*

Case No. 2767:  Alleged Father O   MN  $Rh_2rh$  K neg. S neg.
                Mother          A₁  MN  $Rh_o$    K neg. S neg.
                Child           A₁  MN  $Rh_o$    K pos. S neg.

A child who is **Kell**-positive, must have inherited the gene for the Kell agglutinogen from either of his parents. Since neither the alleged father nor the mother are **Kell**-positive, paternity is excluded.

*Duffy Exclusions*

Case No. 2647:  Alleged Father O MN  $Rh_1rh$   K neg. Fy(a–b+)
                Mother          A N   $Rh_2rh$   K neg. Fy(a–b–)
                Child           A MN  $Rh_1Rh_2$ K neg. Fy(a+b–)

A child who is **Fy**(a+) must at least have one parent who possesses this factor. Since neither the alleged father nor the mother are **Fy**(a+), paternity is excluded. Exclusion based on the test for Duffy factors must be corroborated and controlled carefully. Until substantial statistical family study is available, the results of such findings can only be offered as presumptive evidence.

*Multiple Exclusions*

Case No. 2747:  Alleged Father  $A_1$  M  $Rh_1rh$  K neg.  S pos.
Mother                O   N  $Rh_1rh$  K neg.  S pos.
Child                 O   N  $Rh_1Rh_2$ K neg.  S pos.

There is a double exclusion of paternity present.
1. A child of type N cannot have a father of type M ($M^g$ neg.).
2. A child who is **rh''**-positive (phenotype $Rh_2$) must have inherited the gene for **rh''** from either of his parents. Since neither the alleged father nor the mother have this factor, paternity is excluded.

Case No. 2815:  Alleged Father O  MN  $Rh_o$     K pos.  S neg.
Mother                O   N   $Rh_1rh$  K neg.  S neg.
Child                 O   MN  $Rh_1Rh_2$ K neg.  S pos.

There is a double exclusion of paternity present.
1. A child who is **S**-positive must have inherited the gene for S from either of his parents.
2. A child who is **rh''**-positive must have inherited the gene for the **rh''** from either of his parents. Since the alleged father and the mother are S-negative as well as **rh''**-negative, there is a double exclusion of paternity.

Case No. 2643:  Alleged Father  B    MN   $Rh_o$     K neg.
Mother                O    MN   $Rh_1rh$   K neg.
Child                 $A_2$   N   $Rh_1Rh_2$  K pos.

There is a triple exclusion of paternity present:
1. A child of group A must have inherited a gene for the A agglutinogen from either of his parents.
2. A child who is **rh''**-positive must have inher-

ited the gene for **rh″** from either of his parents. 3. A child who is **Kell**-positive must have inherited the gene for **Kell** from either of his parents. Since neither the alleged father nor the mother have the $A_2$ factor, the **rh″** factor, or the **Kell** factor, there is a triple exclusion of paternity.

Case No. 2461:

| | | | | |
|---|---|---|---|---|
| Alleged Father | O | N | $Rh_1Rh_1$ | K neg. |
| Mother | O | MN | $Rh_2rh$ | K neg. |
| Child (Age 15) | O | MN | $Rh_o.$ | K neg. |

Pat. excl. ($Rh_o$)

| | | | | |
|---|---|---|---|---|
| Child (Age 13) | O | N | $Rh_1rh$ | K neg. |

Pat. not excl.

| | | | | |
|---|---|---|---|---|
| Child (Age 10) | O | M | $Rh_2rh$ | K neg. |

Pat. excl. (M)

| | | | | |
|---|---|---|---|---|
| Child (Age 7) | O | M | $Rh_2Rh_2$ | K neg. |

Pat. excl. (M + $Rh_2$)

| | | | | |
|---|---|---|---|---|
| Child (Age 3) | O | M | $Rh_1Rh_2$ | K neg. |

Pat. excl. (M)

| | | | | |
|---|---|---|---|---|
| Child (Age 2) | O | MN | $Rh_2rh$ | K neg. |

Pat. excl. (rh)

There are multiple exclusions of paternity involving five of the six children. If the alleged father is the parent of the thirteen-year-old child, then at least two other men must be considered in order to have the variety of blood factors that the six children demonstrate. This is analyzed as follows:

1. The father of the fifteen-year-old child must provide an $R^o$ (or $r$) gene.

2. The father of the thirteen-year-old child must provide an $R^1$ (or $r'$) and $N$ gene.

3. The father of the ten-year-old child must provide an $R^2$ (or $r''$) or $R^o$ (or $r$) and an $M$ gene.

4. The father of the seven-year-old child must provide an $R^2$ (or $r''$) and $M$ gene.

5. The father of the three-year-old child must provide an $R^1$ (or $r'$) and $M$ gene.

6. The father of the two-year-old child must provide an $R^2$ ( or $r''$ ) or $R^o$ (or $r$) gene.

Since one father cannot provide more than two Rh genes, it would require at least two fathers to supply the needed $R^o$, $R^1$, $R^2$, and $r$ genes that the six children possess. In addition, if there were only two fathers involved, they would have to be of genotype *MN* $R^1r$ and *MN* $R^2R^o$ in order to supply the combination of genes these six children possess. And neither of these genotypes is the genotype of the alleged father! The most charitable conclusion is that the alleged father is the parent of the child, age thirteen, and that two other men fathered the other five children.

The finding of an exclusion in more than one blood group system is not unusual but does not carry any greater significance than does a single exclusion. An argument frequently presented by attorneys questions the validity of a single exclusion in one blood group system, while several other blood groups fail to exclude. This line of reasoning neglects the fact that many of the characteristics of humans may be similar, but that no characteristic can begin *de novo*—each characteristic must be inherited from a parent. Thus, a blood factor cannot be present in the blood of a child unless present in the mother or the father. Any *single* inheritable characteristic is the basis for an exclusion of parentage if it cannot be accounted for by the established laws of heredity.

## IDENTIFICATION AND REPORT FORMS

The final report submitted to the courts must decisively indicate, clearly and without confusion, the conclusion of the expert who performed the test. A uniform form does not exist; most experts devise their own model. The essential facts should indicate:

1. The methods of identification of the persons tested—mutual identification, pictures of the persons, signatures, and fingerprinting are the usual methods.
2. The individual tests used and the results of these tests—

REPORT ON

BLOOD GROUPING TEST

IN THE MATTER OF

Docket No._____

_____against_____

Pursuant to an order duly entered in the above entitled action,
I proceeded to examine the following named persons on the dates
listed below:

| DATE | NAME | IDENTIFICATION |
|------|------|----------------|
|      |      |                |
|      |      |                |
|      |      |                |

Figure 8-1

Date_____

Clerk of the Family Court
County of Kings
283 Adams Street
Brooklyn, New York

RE:_____VS:_____

Docket No._____

Gemtlemen:

I am herewith submitting results of blood tests performed
on _____(alleged father),_____(mother),and
_____(child) in reference to paternity dispute on the
above case.

Results of the blood tests follow:

|                       |         |    | $Rh_o$ | rh' | rh'' | hr' | hr'' | S | K |           |
|-----------------------|---------|----|------|-----|-----|-----|-----|---|---|-----------|
| (alleged father)      | $A_1$   | M  | +    | -   | +   | +   | -   | + | - | $Rh_2Rh_2$ |
| (mother)              | $A_1$   | N  | +    | +   | -   | +   | +   | + | - | $Rh_1rh$   |
| (child)               | $A_1$   | MN | +    | -   | +   | +   | +   | + | - | $Rh_2rh$   |

There are no contradictions to the laws of theoretical expectancy
in these findings: paternity therefore cannot be excluded.

Respectfully submitted,

Leon N. Sussman, M.D.

Figure 8-2

Date_____

Mr. London, Esq.
Clerk of the Family Court
135 East 22nd Street
New York, N.Y.

RE:_____(putative father)

_____(mother)

_____(child)

Docket No._____

Dear Mr. London:

I am herewith submitting results of blood tests performed on
_____(alleged father),_____(mother), and
_____(child) in reference to paternity dispute on the above
case.

Results of the blood tests follow:

|  | | Rh$_o$ | rh' | rh" | hr' | hr" | S | K | |
|---|---|---|---|---|---|---|---|---|---|
| (alleged father) | O N | + | + | - | - | + | - | - | Rh$_1$Rh$_1$ |
| (mother) | A$_1$ MN | + | + | - | + | + | + | - | Rh$_1$rh |
| (child) | A$_1$ M | + | + | - | + | + | - | - | Rh$_1$rh |

There is a contradiction to the laws of theoretical expectancy,
in that a father of group N must transmit an N factor to his child.
Since the putative father,_____, is group N and the child,____,
is group M (lacking the N factor), paternity is therefore excluded.

Very truly yours,

Leon N. Sussman, M.D.

Figure 8-3

the results of subgrouping, other blood grouping tests,
titrations, and scoring (if performed) should be reported.
Control tests, which are always performed, are included
in the report by some workers.

3. The final conclusion and the basis for these conclusions—
although not usually included in the official report, all
tests are done in duplicate, using different lots of testing
serums. In the event of an exclusion, retesting of the sample is done. In some cases, the entire tests are repeated
after obtaining fresh specimens and may even be sent to

another expert for confirmation. These details need not be part of the official report, which should be kept as simple as possible. They should, however, form part of the laboratory record and be available if requested. The identification and report form used by the author is a simplified one that can be easily understood by the laity. (Figs. 8-1, 8-2, and 8-3).

## THE QUALIFIED EXPERT

The expert in the performance of blood grouping tests, whose qualifications have been outlined by the Committee on Medico-legal Problems of the AMA,[29] should be expected to defend his conclusions on the witness stand. He must also be prepared to give proper and satisfactory answers to questions based on the following, which were originally asked by Schatkin:[8]

1. Were the proper methods and techniques employed in arriving at the exclusion?
2. Were fresh, potent serums used, and were the blood specimens and parties properly identified?
3. Was the serologist fully qualified and his integrity beyond question?
4. Was the test accurate and reliable, with all possibility of error ruled out?
5. Has the serologist, testifying under cross-examination in support of the exclusion, successfully withstood attack on his skill and integrity, techniques employed, identification of parties and blood specimens, and complete accuracy and reliability of the test?

To neglect to perform at least three usually accepted blood grouping tests in all matters where paternity is an issue is to deny the courts the most effective means of resolving the question. The falsely accused man may be deprived of a defense that can exonerate him 53 percent of the time. Even if the man admits paternity, his belief that he is the father could be erroneous. A blood test analysis that can be performed quickly may decisively change the entire aspect of a case. Thus, no paternity case should be permitted to proceed to final judgment until the results of the blood grouping tests have been considered.

Although the number of qualified experts may be limited, the availability of air transportation makes them easily accessible. In an exclusion where the results are questioned, the submission of the blood samples to another independent expert will be supportive. This corroboration is an essential step in justifying the report of an exclusion.

The contribution to forensic medicine made by the use of results obtained by blood grouping tests is a considerable one. Their accuracy, reliability, and validity are such that the help of the experts in this field should be consulted in all questions involving filial relationships.

## REFERENCES

1. Neil, J. V.: The study of human mutation rates. *Amer. Nat.*, 86:129, 1952.
2. Haselhorst, G., and Lauer, A.: Uber eine Blutgruppenkombination Mutter AB und Kind O. *Ztschr. f.d. ges. Anat.*, 15:205, 1930.
3. Sussman, L. N.: Blood grouping tests. Application to related scientific fields. *Am. J. Med. Tech.*, March-April, 1965, p. 87.
4. Wiener, A. S., and Leff, I. L.: Chances of establishing the non-identity of bi-ovular twins. *Genetics*, 25:187, 1940.
5. Smith, S. M., and Penrose, L. S.: Monozygotic and dizygotic twin diagnosis. *Ann. Human Genet.*, 19:273, 1955.
6. Walsh, R. J., and Kooptzoff, O.: A study of twins. Blood groups and other data. *Aust. J. Exper. Biol. & M. Sci.*, 33:189, 1955.
7. Race, R. R., and Sanger, R.: *Blood Groups in Man.* 4th ed. Philadelphia, F. A. Davis Co., 1962, p. 369.
8. Schatkin, S. B.: *Disputed Paternity Proceedings.* 4th ed. New York, Mathew Bender & Co., 1967.
9. Committee on Medico-Legal Problems of the American Medical Association—Owen, R. D., Stormont, C., Wexler, I. B., and Wiener, A. S.: Medicolegal application of blood grouping tests. *J.A.M.A.*, 164:2036, 1957.
10. Wiener, A. S.: Application of blood grouping tests in cases of disputed maternity. *J. Forensic Sci.*, 4:351, 1959.
11. Shatkin, S. B., Sussman, L. N., and Yarbrough, D. E.: Blood test evidence to detect false claims of citizenship. *New York Law Journal*, 133:110, 1955.

12. Sussman, L. N.: Application of blood grouping to derivative citizenship. *J. Forensic Sci., 1:*101, 1956.
13. Wiener, A. S., and Sonn, E. B.: Heredity of the Rh blood types: IV. Medicolegal application in cases of disputed parentage. *J. Lab. & Clin. Med., 30:*395, 1945.
14. Alvarez, J. de J.: Exclusion de paternidad par medio de los grupos A, B, y O, los factores M y N, los subtipos de Rh y el Hr. *Bol. Asoc. med Santiago, 6:*463, 1948.
15. Unger, L. J.: Blood grouping tests for exclusion of paternity. *J.A.M.A., 152:*1006, 1953.
16. Sussman, L. N.: Blood grouping tests in disputed paternity proceedings. *J.A.M.A., 155:*1143, 1954.
17. Sussman, L. N.: Blood grouping tests in disputed paternity proceedings and filial relationship. *J. Forensic Sci., 1:*25, 1956.
18. Wiener, A. S.: Blood grouping tests in disputed parentage. *J. Forensic Sci. Med., 3:*139, 1956.
19. Sussman, L. N.: Survey of paternity disputes in New York City. *J. Forensic Sci., 4:*448, 1959.
20. Marsters, R. W.: Determination of non-paternity by blood groups. *J. Forensic Sci., 2:*15, 1957.
21. Andresen, P. H.: Reliability of the exclusion of paternity after the MN and ABO systems as elucidated by 20,000 mother-child examinations and its significance to the medicolegal conclusion. *Acta Path. et Microbiol. Scandinav., 24:*543, 1947.
22. Orth, G. W., and Hirth, L.: Statistische Untersuchungen in 1341 Paternitäts-prozessen über die Bedeutung der Rh-Untertypen. *Deutsche Ztschr. ges. gerichtl. Med., 42:*270, 1953.
23. Barandun, S., Bühler, W., Hässig, A. and Rosin, S.: Uber die Verwendung der Blutgruppenmerkmale Kell und Duffy[a] zur Klärung von strittigen Abstammungs-fragen. *Med. Prob. Ped., 1:*654, 1954.
24. Henningsen, K.: On the application of blood group testing to cases of disputed paternity in Denmark. *Acta Med. Leg. Soc., 9:*95, 1956.
25. Race, R. R., and Sanger, R.: *Blood Groups in Man.* 5th ed. Philadelphia, F. A. Davis Co., 1962, p. 459.
26. Sussman, L. N.: Blood grouping tests. A review of 1,000 cases of disputed paternity. *Am. J. Clin. Path., 40:*38, 1963.
27. Sussman, L. N., and Schatkin, S. B.: Blood grouping tests in undisputed paternity proceedings. *J.A.M.A., 164:*249, 1957.
28. Schatkin, S. B., and Sussman, L. N.: Blood tests as a prerequisite to commencement of paternity proceedings. *New York Law Journal, 137:*March 19, 1957.
29. Davidsohn, I., Levine, P., and Wiener, A. S.: Medicolegal application of blood grouping tests. *J.A.M.A., 149:*699, 1952.

# CHAPTER NINE

# SUPPLEMENTARY APPLICATIONS

Leon N. Sussman

CRIMINOLOGISTS, anthropologists, geneticists, and other scientific groups have used the information obtained from blood grouping tests in their investigations. Ingenious workers have demonstrated the usefulness of these tests in many areas such as the mapping of chromosomes,[1] the explanation of infertility[2] and miscarriages,[3] the understanding of immunological tolerance, and the association of blood groups with disease.[4] Some of these areas are still controversial, but a brief description of how blood grouping tests have been used in these fields is of interest.

## IDENTIFICATION OF BLOOD SPECIMENS AND BLOOD STAINS

In criminalistics, the ability to exclude a suspect as the source of a submitted blood specimen or a blood stain may be of extreme value. Murder, assault, and accidents such as "hit and run" injuries are situations where blood testing can be helpful. Again, it must be emphasized that these results have solely a *negative* value—the tests can only prove that the sample is *not* the blood of the suspect. Experts qualified in this field must be especially trained and experienced since the identification procedures are fraught with pitfalls and the conclusions have serious consequences. The Federal Bureau of Investigation in Washington, D. C. maintains special facilities for this type of work and may be consulted for advice.

The first step in such studies consists of identifying the specimen as blood. Dyes and paint, especially in the presence of contamination, dirt, and other organic materials frequently resemble blood. The usual method to identify the presence of hemoglobin is a chemical test, utilizing the benzidine or phenolphthalein reactions.

Having established the material as most likely blood, the next step is to prove the specimen is *human* blood. The microscopic appearance of human blood is well known. Any deviation in the appearance of blood cells, such as unusual size and shape, or the presence of nucleated red cells, or ring-shaped nuclei in the leukocytes suggest animal origin. A very sensitive precipitin test, which is species-specific, can be used for positive identification of material of human origin though the antiserums cross-react with nonhuman primate blood. This is an excellent test for soluble material and can be performed in most immunological laboratories.

The determination of the specific blood groups of the specimen depends on the condition of the sample. Fresh blood stains or clots can be suspended in saline and examined by the usual methods as described for the blood grouping tests. A complete grouping, utilizing the many blood systems, can thus be done and a thorough comparison made between the sample and the blood of the suspect. Old blood stains and blood crusts present much more difficult problems. The fragile red blood cells are usually quickly hemolyzed, thus preventing the direct identification of their agglutinogens. The agglutinins present may be preserved in the stain and can occasionally be identified. However, the most successful method involves the ability of the blood group substance in the clot or stain to absorb the agglutinins in a testing serum of known titer. Meticulous care is necessary to assure that this absorption is specific for blood since body secretions such as sweat or saliva can also absorb the agglutinins, thus giving misleading results. The test must be controlled by the simultaneous testing of an adjacent nonbloodstained sample which has been similarly exposed, soiled, or otherwise contaminated. Under favorable conditions, the A-B-O grouping may be determined on old clots and stains. (A very thorough description of the technics is outlined in Chapter Two.) Sometimes the M agglutinogen can also be identified. The other blood group agglutinogens cannot be reliably determined in old blood stains. The subject has been thoroughly studied by Wiener, who has had extensive experience in these areas as Serologist to the Office of the Chief Medical Examiner of the City of New York.[5]

## Case 1

A recent "mugging" murder of an elderly man was investigated. Death resulted from numerous stab wounds with spattering of blood over the clothes of both the victim and his assailant. In the assault, the attacker's hand was cut. A trail of his blood through the snow led police to him. Of particular interest were the blood stains found on the gloves in the assailant's possession when he was apprehended. Some of the stains were group O, corresponding to the victim's blood group, and others were group B, corresponding to the blood group of the murderer.* After this evidence was presented, the defendant was found guilty.

## Case 2

A truck was suspected of being involved in a "hit and run" accident in which a pedestrian was killed. Such vehicles are routinely examined by the police department for evidence of blood stains or bits of human tissue. While inspecting the chassis and tires of the truck, the police found a small red stain between the treads of the recently washed tires. The entire tire was brought to the laboratory where the stain was extracted and proven to be human blood. Blood grouping tests could not be performed because of the small size of the specimen. However, the identification of the stain as human blood was sufficient to obtain an admission from the driver concerning the accident.*

## Case 3

In 1955, a defendant was convicted and sentenced to death for the rape-murder of an eight-year-old child. A major factor in the conviction was the testimony of the prosecutor's expert. He identified the "reddish" stains on a pair of shorts found in the suspect's apartment as human blood of group A, corresponding to the blood group of the child. The prisoner's blood group was O. The defendant's attorney was denied permission for an

---

* A. S. Wiener, personal communication.

independent analysis of the "blood stained shorts" until 1963. During the eight intervening years the shorts were in a metal locker in the custody of the Court. The examination in 1963 failed to reveal any evidence that the "stains" were blood. Tests for hemoglobin by chemical and spectroscopic methods were entirely negative. Microanalysis of fibers obtained from the stained areas revealed crystalline mineral particles identified as paint. The question was then raised as to the methods that had originally been used for the identification of the stains as human blood of Group A. On the basis of these new findings the Supreme Court of the United States reversed the conviction and ordered the prisoner released.

IDENTIFICATION OF BLOOD GROUPS BY STUDY OF THE SECRETIONS: The subject of group specific substances in the body secretions was investigated in 1930.[6] The early researchers soon recognized that the ability to secrete these substances was a genetically determined trait that obeyed the Mendelian law of inheritance.[7, 8] This characteristic was present in 80 percent of Caucasians. They were called secretors and designated as bearers of the gene *Se*. The 20 percent of Caucasians who were nonsecretors lacked this gene and were designated as *se*. The presence of the group specific substance in a secretion of the body can be demonstrated by its ability to inhibit the normal agglutinating activity of an antiserum with the appropriate red blood cells. Thus, the saliva of an A secretor when mixed with anti-**A** serum would prevent the agglutination of A cells by the serum. The saliva of a nonsecretor has no such inhibitory effect. This test is easily done with anti-**A** or anti-**B** serum for group A, B, or AB subjects. The group O secretors can not be identified in this manner since anti-**O** does not exist. This problem was resolved by the finding that the lectin derived from the seeds of *Ulex Europaeus* could separate secretors and nonsecretors of all blood groups.[9, 10] This specificity is called anti-**H**.[11] The reaction is strong with O and $A_2$ bloods, less with $A_1$ and B bloods and least with $A_1B$ bloods. The exact status of the H substance is not clearly defined. It is considered by some to be the precursor of the A-B-O substance;[12] others are of the opinion that the *H* gene and the *A-B-O* genes compete for the same substrate to produce either H or A-B-O substance.[13]

Landsteiner and Levine[14] had previously demonstrated the presence of A and B substance in tissue cells, such as liver and kidney. This new field, therefore, permits the identification of the A-B-O blood group in about 80 percent of Caucasians by examination of the saliva, sweat, gastric juice, tears, stool, and urine. The examination of body tissue such as stomach, pancreas, gland, liver, and even bones can also reveal the blood grouping. Of particular interest is the paper describing the blood groupings determined on the bones and muscles of 300 Egyptian mummies (circa 3000 B.C.) by Boyd and Boyd.[15]

The inhibition technic is the method of choice for the determination of the blood groups when examining secretions and body tissues. Numerous sensitive quantitative methods have been described for these tests.[16] Careful laboratory procedures with constant controls are necessary to assure the specific nature of the reaction. Especially to be questioned are conclusions based on the *failure* to inhibit, since the substance that was originally present may have deteriorated, thus giving negative reactions. The reader is again referred to Chapter Two for more details.

Several criminal cases have been solved as the result of tests performed on body secretions. The determination of the blood groups from seminal stains on clothing, saliva on cigarette butts, nasal secretions or sputum on handkerchiefs, and stains of other body secretions on various objects have been introduced as evidence.[17] The exclusion of a suspect by comparison between his blood group and that of the incriminating blood stains or body secretion can indeed be a major element in defense.

## Case 4

The body of a woman was found in the street. She had been strangled and two knotted men's handkerchiefs were nearby. Saline extracts of the handkerchief revealed human secretion of group B. The victim was group A. The suspect who had been seen carrying the body was group B. Stains on the linoleum of his room were examined. These proved to be of human origin, evidently saliva or edema fluid as a result of strangulation. They were of group A, corresponding to the deceased's blood grouping. The accused confessed when presented with these findings.

It must again be emphasized that such blood grouping tests on dried blood, old clots, blood stains, and body secretion stains should be performed only in laboratories where experts with the necessary skill, experience, and knowledge can perform and interpret these tests and thus arrive at valid conclusions.

## BLOOD GROUPS AND DISEASE

A considerable literature has developed attempting to associate the blood groups with increased susceptibility to various diseases. The report in 1953 linking cancer of the stomach with blood group A has been corroborated, reviewed, then refuted, and even denied by different authors. Other associations such as group O with duodenal ulcer, group A with pernicious anemia and group A with diabetes mellitus, and nonsecretors with duodenal ulcer have been statistically proferred and as frequently contested. Many references to this material can be found in Race and Sanger.[18] Wiener has strongly criticized these results, which he asserts are deduced from improper methods of sampling and other statistical errors.[19]

## BLOOD GROUPS AND ANTHROPOLOGY

The study of the blood group frequencies in various parts of the world had led to interesting theories concerning population drifts, origin of ethnic groups, and certain racial blood group characteristics. One such hypothesis links the finding of the Diego factor in such widely separated cultures as the South American Indians with Asiatic Mongoloids, as evidence of the colonization of the Americas via a land bridge from Siberia to Alaska. Maps of the world illustrating and analyzing the distribution of the blood groups have been constructed by Mourant.[20] Other references to the movements of ancient civilizations and the mixing of populations have been reported by Boyd,[21] Wiener,[22] Simmons,[23] and others.

## BLOOD GROUPS AND GENETICS

The ease with which inherited characteristics can be visually and clearly demonstrated with the red blood cells provides geneticists with a useful tool. The large numbers of family studies which proved that the genes determining the blood groups followed Mendelian laws, quickly established the value of these groups as chromosome markers. This subject was advanced by the discovery in 1962 of the $Xg^a$ blood group system.[24] The statistical proof that $Xg^a$ is a sex-linked gene carried on the X chromosome[25] supplied an important marker in the mapping of this one chromosome.

To date, this mapping has resulted in the approximate localization of the genes determining hemophilia, red-green color blindness, glucose-6-phosphate dehydrogenase deficiency, and a special variety of muscular dystrophy as well as the $Xg^a$ gene–all on the X chromosome. The problem of locating the position of the many other genes on the twenty-three pairs of human chromosomes is a staggering one, but it has begun and must be continued since it is an essential step in the development of the gene theory and the concept of gene modification.

Blood grouping tests have enhanced the administration of justice in many criminal cases. The study of gene localization has been launched with the tentative description of the position of several loci on the X chromosomes. Anthropologists and geneticists have applied blood grouping in their studies. These contributions to related scientific fields have proven to be of great value and will become even greater as more investigators discover newer areas to explore by blood grouping.

## REFERENCES

1. McKusick, V. A.: On the X chromosome of man. *Ann. Int. Med.,* 56:991, 1962.
2. Behrman, S. J., Buettner-Janusch, J., Heglar, R., Gershowitz, H., and Tew, W. L.: ABO (H) blood incompatibility as a cause of infertility: a new concept. *Am. J. Obst. & Gynec.,* 79:847, 1960.
3. Levine, P.: Serological factors as possible causes in spontaneous abortions. *J. Hered.,* 34:71, 1943.

4. Buckwalter, J. A., Wohlwend, E. B., Colter, D. C., Tidrick, R. T. and Knowler, L. A.: ABO blood groups and disease. *J.A.M.A., 162:*1210, 1956.

5. Wiener, A. S., and Gordon, E. B.: Examination of blood stains in forensic medicine. *J. Forensic Sci., 1:*89, 1956.

6. Schiff, F., and Sasaki, H.: Ueber die Vererbung des serologischen Ausscheidungstypus. *Ztschr. f. Immunitatsforsch., 77:*129, 1932.

7. Schiff, F., and Sasaki, H.: Der Ausscheidungstypus, ein auf serologischen Wege nachweisbares mendelndes Merkmal. *Klin. Woch., 34:*1426, 1932.

8. Friedenreich, V., and Hartmann, G.: Ueber die Verteilung der Gruppenantigene im Organismus der sogenannten "Ausscheider" und "Nictausscheider." *Ztschr. f. Immunitatsforsch., 92:*141, 1938.

9. Boyd, W. C., and Shapleigh, E.: Separation of individuals of any blood group into secretors and non-secretors by use of a plant agglutinin (lectin). *Blood, 9:*1195, 1954.

10. Wiener, A. S., Gordon, E. B., and Evans, A.: The value of anti-**H** reagents *(Ulex europaeus)* for grouping dried blood stains. *J. Forensic Sci., 3:*493, 1958.

11. Morgan, W. T. J., and Watkins, W. M.: The detection of a product of the blood group O gene and the relationship of the so-called O substance to the agglutinogens A and B. *Brit. J. Exper. Path., 29:*159, 1948.

12. Watkins, W. M., and Morgan, W. T. J.: Possible genetical pathway for the biosynthesis of blood group mucopolysaccharides. *Vox Sanguinis, 4:*97, 1959.

13. Wiener, A. S., Moor-Jankowski, J., and Gordon, E. B.: The relationship of the H substance to the A-B-O blood groups. *Internat. Arch. Allergy, 29:*82, 1966.

14. Landsteiner, K., and Levine, P.: Group specific substances in spermatozoa. *J. Immunol., 12:*415, 1926.

15. Boyd, W. C., and Boyd, L. G.: Blood grouping tests on 300 mummies. *J. Immunol., 32:*307, 1937.

16. Pretshold, H.: A hemagglutination-inhibition titration technic for detecting and measuring antigen substance specificity in secretor saliva. *Am. J. Med. Tech.,* July-Aug. 1964, p. 236.

17. Wiener, A. S.: Forensic importance of blood grouping. *Exper. Med. & Surg., 2:*44, 1944.

18. Race, R. R., and Sanger, R.: *Blood Groups in Man.* 4th ed. Philadelphia, F. A. Davis Co., 1962, p. 393.

19. Wiener, A. S., and Wexler, I. B.: Blood group paradoxes. *J.A.M.A., 162:*1474, 1956.

20. Mourant, A.: *The Distribution of the Human Blood Groups.* Oxford, Blackwell Scientific Publications, 1954.

21. Boyd, W. C.: Blood groups. *Tabulae Biologicae, 17:*113, 1939.

22. Wiener, A. S.: *Blood Groups and Transfusion.* 3d ed. New York, Hafner Publishing Co., 1943.

23. Simmons, R. T.: A report on blood group genetical surveys in Eastern Asia, Indonesia, Melanesia, Micronesia, Polynesia, and Australia in the study of man. *Anthropos, 51:*500, 1956.

24. Mann, J., Cahan, A., Gelb, A., Fisher, N., Hamper, J., Tippett, P., Sanger, R., and Race, R. R.: A sex-linked blood group. *Lancet, 1:*8, 1962.

25. Wall, R. L., McConnell, J., Moore, D., Macpherson, C. R., and Marson, A.: Christmas disease, color-blindness and blood group Xg[a]. *Am. J. Med., 43:*214, 1967.

CHAPTER TEN

# A PREVIEW OF THE FUTURE
# IN BLOOD GROUPING

Leon N. Sussman

THE ADVANCES in the field of molecular biology, immunology, and automated medical technology has made available a large quantity of data whose impact has not yet been thoroughly explored. Hidden within the vast body of information now being acquired, is the possibility of gene manipulation and modification which has as its goal the elimination of undesirable genes and the traits they determine. This idea evokes many moral and ethical problems that unquestionably will soon be raised and must eventually be faced.

The facts on which any such philosophy is based relate to those studies which expose hereditary characteristics of multiple biological systems. The red blood cell agglutinogens, identified by their many blood factors, are the best known to date. The results of the studies of the inherited groups of the leukocytes, platelets, hemoglobin, and plasma fractions further the hypothesis that there are no exactly similar individuals, except for identical twins.

## BLOOD CELL GROUPS
### The Red Cell Blood Groups

As has been shown, the many combinations of the blood group systems permit the identification of several million individual blood types with the present available antiserums. This does not exhaust all the possibilities, however, since new publications bring to attention still other hitherto unrecognized blood group systems that further extend the table of individual blood types.

### The White Cell (Leukocyte) Blood Groups (H L-A Antigens)

Leukocyte antibodies were first regularly observed in 1953.[1]

162

These were shown to be immune in origin, stimulated either by repeated pregnancies or multiple transfusions. The antigens recognized by these antibodies were shown to be inherited characteristics by studies in twins[2] and by their transmission from father to child.[3, 4] Leuko-agglutinins were found in the serum of 20 percent of multiparous women.[5] These women provided the best testing serums as there was a greater probability that during pregnancy only a single antigenic stimulus provoked the antibody. In multitransfused patients, the presence of many antibodies seriously interfered with clear-cut patterns of inheritance. Several attempts at a nomenclature for this system have been proposed, none of which are universally accepted. Approximately thirty-one leukocyte antigens have already been defined, although evidence for cross-reactions and multiple antibodies continue to confuse the true picture. When these antigens are properly sorted out and when reproducible reactions are demonstrated, a substantial contribution to the science of immunology may be anticipated.[6] The present interest in the blood groups of lymphocytes lies in their relationship to graft rejections—particularly in the study of organ transplantation.[7] (Table 10-I).

TABLE 10-I

THE HL-A ALLELES
(2 Loci on Chromosome #6)

| *First Series* | *Second Series* |
|---|---|
| HL-A1 | HL-A5 |
| HL-A2 | HL-A7 |
| HL-A3 | HL-A8 |
| HL-A9 | HL-A12 |
| W-23 | HL-A13 |
| W-24 | W 5 |
| HL-10 | W 10 |
| W 25 | W 14 |
| W 26 | W 15 |
| HL-A11 | W 16 |
| W 19 | W 17 |
| W 29 | W 18 |
| W 30 | W 21 |
| W 31 | W 22 |
| W 32 | W 27 |
| W 28 | |

## Platelet Blood Group[8]

The difficulty of correctly typing blood platelets is complicated by the tendency of these blood elements to spontaneous agglutination, especially in a coagulation substrate such as plasma or serum.[9] Complex serological techniques involving heat-inactivation and antiglobulin consumption are necessary to avoid misleading results. Platelet antibodies have been studied as etiological agents in thrombocytopenic purpura,[10] neonatal thrombocytopenia,[11] and drug induced purpuras. The antigens A and B of the A-B-O red blood cell system have been identified in platelets.[12] The platelet antibodies are found in the gammaglobulin fractions of the serum, whereas the leukocyte agglutinins are found in the betaglobulin fractions. The difficult problem of typing platelets must still be met, but eventually this system will provide additional means of differentiating between individuals.

## OTHER BLOOD CONSTITUENTS
### Hemoglobin Types

Hemoglobin has been found to have a definite electrophoretic mobility depending upon its electrical charge. This in turn is determined by the amino acid sequence in the polypeptide chains composing the hemoglobin. In 1949, the first demonstration of a hemoglobin electrophoretic pattern differing from normal was noted when sickle-cell hemoglobin was tested.[13] The ability to differentiate between the homozygous SS and the heterozygous AS hemoglobins led to exhaustive studies of this subject. The inheritance of the genes determining sickling was shown to follow the Mendelian rules.[14] Numerous other variants of hemoglobin have been investigated and a nomenclature has developed. These abnormal hemoglobins are designated by the letters of the alphabet (Hgb A to Q) and their subtypes by their place of origin, e.g. Hemoglobin G Singapore. Further refinement of the technic, consisting of electrophoretic chromatography after tryptic digestion, resulted in two-dimensional maps of the individual peptides called "fingerprinting."[15] The complicated subject of hemoglobin electrophoresis is thoroughly reviewed in Miale's Hematology.[16]

Since these uncommon hemoglobins are inherited, they can play a role in parentage, identification, and similar studies.

### Haptoglobin Groups
### (Refer to Chapter Six)

The electrophoresis of serum on starch gel has separated many individual fractions of the plasma proteins.[17] Among these is haptoglobin, an interesting glycoprotein component of the alpha-2-globulin. This protein is capable of combining with free hemoglobin to form a firm complex, thus binding the hemoglobin. Three separate groups of the haptoglobin protein can be differentiated. They have been named type 1-1, type 2-2, and type 2-1. They are easily separated by electrophoretic technics. A rare variant, in which no haptoglobin is found, has also been observed. The genetic control is through a three-gene system, named $IIp^1$, $Hp^2$, and $Hp^0$.[18] The predicted pattern of inheritance has not revealed any exceptions; the system, therefore, could be utilized in studies of parentage. Tables demonstrating the types of haptoglobin that can be expected in the offspring of assorted matings have been published.[19] The gene frequencies were determined in 564 mother-child combinations. The probable exclusion rate for wrongly accused men was calculated as approximately 18 percent.[20] The inclusion of the haptoglobin group analysis in parentage studies in Sweden and other European countries has increased the composite total probable exclusion rate considerably. To date, this type of examination is being applied to such problems in the United States.

### Gm Groups

The highly diluted serum of some patients with rheumatoid arthritis was found to cause the agglutination of Rh-positive cells coated with incomplete (19S) Rh antibody. An inhibitory substance preventing this reaction was discovered in the normal serum of 60 percent of Caucasians. This inhibitory protein was determined by a gene, $Gm^a$, which is inherited as a Mendelian character.[21] Further study revealed that two other allelic genes, $Gm^b$ and $Gm^x$, controlled this system. Tests on 450 families corroborated the heredity nature of this property.[22] Although the tests require a complicated technic, they do reveal a determinable characteristic that can differentiate between individuals. In Norway, where considerable family studies using the three anti-serums, anti-Gm[a], anti-Gm[b], anti-Gm[x], have been reported, the probable exclusion rate for falsely accused fathers has been calculated to be approximately 27 percent.[23] When the reliability of this test in paternity studies has been thoroughly established, a valuable means of genetic identity and filial relationship will be available.

## Gc Groups

Among the more recently discovered inherited blood and serum characters is the one described by Hirschfeld in 1959.[24] This system was demonstrated by immuno-electrophoresis of the alpha-2-globulins of normal serum. Three phenotypes were recognized and family studies indicated they were determined by two co-dominant genes, $Gc^1$ and $Gc^2$.[25] The homozygous phenotypes were designated as Gc1-1 and Gc2-2, and the heterozygote as Gc2-1, thus following the nomenclature adopted for the hapto-globins. The application of this technic to 1,338 paternity cases in the Scandinavian countries yielded a probable exclusion rate of 15.7 percent.[26, 27] Of interest, is the fact that in approximately 80 percent of the exclusions there was also an exclusion in the A-B-O, M-N, Rh-Hr, or Haptoglobin systems. Other European reports have confirmed the reliability of this test.[28] The use of this new system with its significantly high probable exclusion rate in the problems of identification and genetic relationship is further increasing the composite chance of exonerating a falsely accused defendant.

## OTHER INHERITABLE BLOOD SYSTEMS

A considerable number of other blood cell or plasma systems that can differentiate between individuals have been superficially explored. Large numbers of family studies, the determination of the frequency of exceptions, and the evidence for the reliability and reproducibility of the tests must be carefully evaluated before such systems can be accepted in problems of filial relationship.

One system, the transferrins, which is involved in the intravascular transportation of iron has been shown to have eight separate inheritable forms.[29, 30] Studies with other plasma proteins and enzyme systems that are genetically controlled hold similar possibilities. Their eventual elaboration can be expected to have a significant impact in increasing the number of individuals that can be differentiated.

### Composite Exclusion Rate

The formula for the calculation of the chance of excluding a falsely accused man in a paternity case by multiple blood group system examinations has been prepared by Wiener.[31]

$$P = 1 - (1 - P_1)(1 - P_2)(1 - P_3)\ldots\ldots$$

Where P = The composite probability of exclusion

$P_1$ = the probability of exclusion in one system
$P_2$ = the probability of exclusion in the second system
$P_3$ = the probability of exclusion in the third system, etc.

The chance of exonerating a falsely accused man will vary with the frequency of each of the blood groups in the general population and with the blood groups of the individual man. Among Caucasians, the approximate chance of exclusion in the several systems discussed is as follows:

| | |
|---|---|
| A-B-O | = 20% |
| M-N-S-s | = 31.6% |
| Rh-Hr | = 25% |
| Kell | = 4% |
| Duffy | = 7% |
| Kidd | = 6% |
| Lutheran | = 3.5% |
| Haptoglobin | = 18% |
| Gm | = 27% |
| Gc | = 16% |

Applying these figures to the above formula

$$P = 1 - (1 - .18)(1 - .24)(1 - .25)(1 - .04)(1 - .18)$$
$$(1 = .27)(1 - .16)$$

$$\therefore P = 1 - .238 = 76.2\%$$
$$P = 1 - (1 - .20)(1 - .316)(1 - .25)(1 - .04)(1 - .07)$$
$$(1 - .06)(1 - .035)(1 - .18)(1 - .27)(1 - .16)$$
$$P = 1 - 16.7 = 83.3\%$$

Thus, the present probable exclusion rate in the United States, using only the generally accepted A-B-O, M-N, Rh-Hr systems is about 53 percent, whereas with the use of the other available or soon to be available newer systems, a probable exclusion rate of 83.3 percent can be attained. The incorporation of these more advanced testing technics including the haptoglobin, Gm, and Gc systems will be a decided advantage in parentage and identification problems. The HL-A system will do even more.[32]

It has already been shown that the red cell factors alone can differentiate approximately 57,000,000 different individuals. This figure can now be multiplied by the number of factors that are present in each of the newly discovered systems. The number of different types of individuals would be of such magnitude as to preclude the possibility of "doubles" except for identical twins. Thus, the prophecy of Karl Landsteiner that the blood groups will eventually prove the individuality of every person is well on the way to complete fulfillment.

## REFERENCES

1. Dausset, J., and Nenna, A.: Presence d'une leuco-agglutinine dans trois serums de malades leucopéniques. *Sang., 24:*410, 1953.
2. Lalezari, P., and Spaet, T. H.: Studies on the genetics of leukocyte antigens. *Blood, 14:*748, 1959.
3. Payne, R., and Rolfs, M. R.: Fetomaternal leukocyte incompatibility. *J. Clin. Invest., 37:*1756, 1958.
4. Rood, J. J. van, Leeuwen, A. van, and Bosch, L. J.: *Proc. VIII Cong. Eur. Soc. Hemat.* 1961.
5. Rood, J. J. van, Leeuwen, A. van, and Eernisse, J. G.: Leucocyte antibodies in sera of pregnant women. *Vox Sanguinis, 4:*427, 1959.
6. Payne, R., and Hackel, E.: Inheritance of human leukocyte antigens. *Amer. J. Human Genet., 13:*306, 1961.
7. Silvers, W. K., and Billingham, R. E.: The tissue typing and lymphocyte problems in transplantation immunity. *Med. Clin. N.A., 49:*1661, 1965.

8. Marsh, W. L., Queen, R., Nichols, M. E., and Charles, H.: Studies of MNSsU antigen activity on leukocytes and platelets. *Transfusion, 14:*462, 1974.

9. Tullis, J. L.: Leukocyte and thrombocyte antibodies. *J.A.M.A., 180:*958, 1962.

10. Tullis, J. L.: Platelet antibody tests in the diagnosis of purpura. *New England J. Med., 249:*591, 1953.

11. Shulman, N. R., Aster, R. H., Pearson, A., and Hiller, M. C.: Immunoreactions involving platelets. VI. Reactions of maternal isoantibodies responsible for neonatal purpura. Differentiation of a second platelet antigen system. *J. Clin. Invest., 41:*1059, 1962.

12. Dausset, J., and Malinvaud, G.: Normal and pathological platelet agglutinins investigated by means of shaking method. Confirmation of presence of A and B antigens in platelets. *Vox Sanguinis, 4:*204, 1954.

13. Pauling, L., Itano, H. A., Singer, S. J., and Wells, I. C.: Sickle cell anemia, a molecular disease. *Science, 110:*543, 1949.

14. Neel, J. V.: The inheritance of the sickling phenomenon, with particular reference to sickle cell disease. *Blood, 6:*389, 1951.

15. Ingram, V. M.: Biochemical genetics at a molecular level. *Am. J. Med., 34:*674, 1963.

16. Miale, J. B.: *Laboratory Medicine—Hematology.* 3d ed. St. Louis, C. V. Mosby Co., 1967, p. 750.

17. Smithies, O., and Walker, N.: Genetic control of some serum proteins in normal humans. *Nature, 176:*1265, 1955.

18. Giblett, E. R.: Haptoglobin: a review. *Vox Sanguinis, 6:*513, 1961.

19. Smithies, O., Connell, G. E., and Dixon, G. H.: Inheritance of haptoglobin subtypes. *Am. J. Human Genet., 14:*14, 1962.

20. Beckman, L., Heiken, A., and Hirschfeld, J.: Frequency of haptoglobin types in the Swedish population. *Hereditas, 47:*599, 1961.

21. Grubb, R., and Laurell, A. B.: Hereditary serological human serum groups. *Acta Path. et Microbiol. Scand., 39:*390, 1956.

22. Grubb, R.: *Hereditary gammaglobulin groups in man.* Ciba Foundation Symposium on the Biochemistry of Human Genetics. London, Churchill, 1959, p. 246.

23. Harboe, M., and Lundevall, J.: The application of the Gm system in paternity cases. *Vox Sanguinis, 6:*257, 1961.

24. Hirschfeld, J.: Immuno-electrophoretic demonstration of qualitative differences in human sera and their relation to the haptoglobins. *Acta Path. et Microbiol. Scand., 47:*160, 1959.

25. Hirschfeld, J., Jonsson, B., and Rasmuson, M.: Inheritance of a new group-specific system demonstrated in normal human sera by

means of an immuno-electrophoretic technique. *Nature, 185:*931, 1960.

26. Hirschfeld, J., and Heiken, A.: Application of the Gc system in paternity cases. *Am. J. Human Genet., 15:*19, 1963.
27. Reinskou, T.: Application of the Gc system in 1,338 paternity cases. *Vox Sanguinis, 11:*59, 1966.
28. Reinskou, T.: On the confidence of Gc type determinations. *Vox Sanguinis, 11:*70,1966.
29. Smithies, O., and Connell, G. E.: *Biochemical aspects of the inherited variations in human serum haptoglobins and transferrins.* Ciba Foundation Symposium on the Biochemistry of Human Genetics. London, Churchill, 1959, p. 178.
30. Smithies, O., and Hiller, O.: The genetic control of transferrins in humans. *Biochem. J., 72:*121, 1959.
31. Wiener, A. S., and Wexler, I. B.: *Heredity of the Blood Groups.* New York, Grune & Stratton, 1958, p. 121.
32. Perkins, H. A.: Tissue Typing. *Wadley Medical Bulletin,* 5, no. 2:165, 1975.

## SUGGESTED BIBLIOGRAPHY

American Association of Blood Banks: *Technical Methods and Procedures of the American Association of Blood Banks.* 4th ed. Chicago, Twentieth Century Press, 1966.
Boorman, Kathleen E., and Dodd, Barbara E.: *An Introduction to Blood Group Serology.* 3d ed. Boston, Little, Brown & Co., 1966.
Erskine, Addine G.: *The Principles and Practice of Blood Grouping.* St. Louis, C. V. Mosby Co., 1973.
Miale, John B.: *Laboratory Medicine—Hematology.* 3d ed. St. Louis, C. V. Mosby Co., 1967.
Mollison, P. L.: *Blood Transfusion in Clinical Medicine.* 4th ed. Philadelphia, F. A. Davis Co.
Polesky, H., et al.: *Paternity Testing.* ASCP, 1975.
Prokop, O., and Uhlenbruck, C.: *Lehrbuch der Blut-und-Serum-gruppen.* 2d ed. Leipzig, East Germany, George Thieme, 1963.
Race, R. R. and Sanger, Ruth: *Blood Groups in Man.* 6th ed. Philadelphia, F. A. Davis Co.
Ranganathan, K. S.: *Essentials of Blood Grouping and Clinical Applications.* Madras, India, Jupiter Press Private Limited, 1967.
Schatkin, S.: *Disputed Paternity Proceedings.* 4th ed. New York, Mathew Bender & Co., 1967.
Wiener, A. S.: *Blood Groups and Transfusion.* 3d ed. 1943. Reprinted New York and London, Hafner Publishing Company, 1961.

Wiener, A. S.: *Rh-Hr Blood Types. Applications in Clinical and Legal Medicine and Anthropology.* New York, Grune & Stratton, 1954.

Wiener, A. S., and Wexler, I. B.: *Heredity of Blood Groups.* New York, Grune & Stratton, 1958.

Wiener, A. S.: *Advances in Blood Grouping.* New York, Grune & Stratton, 1961.

Wiener, A. S., and Wexler, I. B.: *Rh-Hr Syllabus.* 2d ed. New York, Grune & Stratton, 1963.

Wiener, A. S., and Shapiro, M.: *Advances in Blood Grouping.* Vol. 2, New York, Grune & Stratton, 1965.

# AUTHOR INDEX

# SUBJECT INDEX

## A

A blood group, 3, 38
*AA*, 13
A₁, 23, 30, 34
A₁B, 23
A₂, 23, 24, 30, 37
A₂B, 23, 24, 37, 38
A₃, 23, 24, 30, 31
A₃B, 24
A₄, 23, 31
Aₑ₁, 23
Aₘ, 23
AB blood group, 3, 26
A-B-O blood group, 8, 9, 13, 16, 21-44, 39
    testing, 27-31
Absorption-elution technic, 42
ACD anticoagulant, 35, 97
Acid Phosphatase (acP), 97, 100, 115
    phenotyping, 99
Acriflavine, 36
Adenosine deaminase (ADA), 100, 103
Adenylate kinase (AK), 100, 103
Agammaglobulinemia, 34
Agglutination, 3, 12, 22, 28, 29, 30, 32, 34, 36, 59, 164
Agglutinins, 25
    cold, 28, 34, 37
Agglutinogens, 10, 11, 12, 13, 14, 66, 67, 76, 89, 91, 154, 162
Alanine aminotransferase, 100
Albumin, 36, 106, 108, 113
    Naskapi, 106
Allele, 3-4, 9
    multiple theory, 66, 70
Alpha methyl dopa, 36
Alpha-2-globulins, 166
Alsever's solution, 35, 97
Am marker, 108
AMP phosphotransferase, 100

Anti-**A**, 3, 12, 13, 14, 22, 23, 24, 27, 28, 30, 31, 32, 33, 34, 35, 37, 41
Anti-AB, 27, 28, 30, 25
Anti-**B**, 3, 12, 14, 22, 25, 27, 28, 31, 32, 33, 34, 41
Anti-antigen, 12 (*see also* Antibody)
Antibody, 12, 69
    cold, 89
    low titer, 34
    placenta transfer, 33
Antigen, 12-13, 21
    acquired, 35
    strong, 12
    weak, 35
Antiglobulin, 164
    test, 36, 69, 71, 76
Anti-Gmᵃ, 166
Anti-Gmᵇ, 166
Anti-Gmᵇ, 166
Anti-Gmˣ, 166
Anti-**H**, 14, 27, 31, 41, 156
Anti-hr′, 64
Anti-hrˢ, 71
Antihuman globulin, 12, 59, 77, 78, 87
Anti-**M**, 4, 12, 13, 49, 56, 57, 60
    dosage, 58
Anti-Mᵏ, 57
Anti-**N**, 4, 12, 13, 49, 56, 57, 60
    dosage, 58
Anti-O, 13
Anti-**Rh**, 63
Anti-rh′, 72
Anti-rhᴳ, 72
Anti-**Rh**₀, 69, 70, 72
Anti-**s**, 51, 57, 59, 60
    dosage, 58
Anti-**S**, 51, 57, 59, 60
    dosage, 58
Antisera, 12, 13, 27 (*see also specific* antigens)
    contaminated, 37